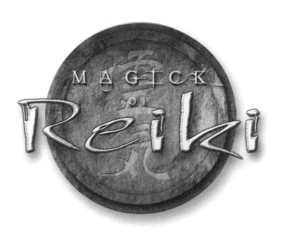

MAGICK
of
Reiki

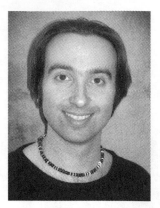

About the Author

Christopher Penczak (New Hampshire) teaches classes throughout New England on witchcraft, meditation, Reiki, crystals, and shamanic journeys in addition to being a part-time faculty member at the North Eastern Institute of Whole Health in New Hampshire. He is a regular presenter, and has been the keynote speaker at the New England Reiki Conference. He is the author of several books, including *The Inner Temple of Witchcraft, The Outer Temple of Witchcraft,* and *The Witch's Shield.*

Focused Energy for Healing, Ritual & Spiritual Development

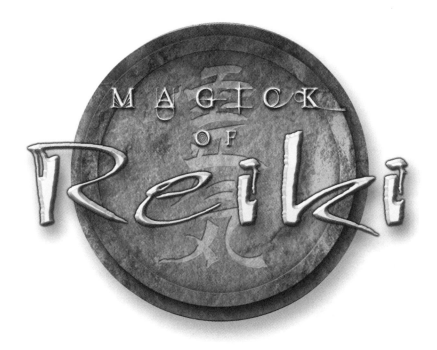

MAGICK
OF
Reiki

CHRISTOPHER PENCZAK

Llewellyn Publications
Woodbury, Minnesota

First Edition
Eighteenth Printing, 2022

Book design by Donna Burch
Background cover image © PhotoDisc.com
Cover design by Kevin R. Brown
Edited by Andrea Neff
Interior Reiki hand position illustrations in chapter three and figure drawings © 2004 by Wendy Froshay
Interior Reiki symbols by Llewellyn art department

Penczak, Christopher.
    Magick of Reiki: focused energy for healing, ritual & spiritual development / Christopher Penczak.—1st ed.
        p.   cm.
    Includes bibliographical references (p.)
    ISBN 13: 978-0-7387-0573-6
    ISBN 10: 0-7387-0573-X
      1. Reiki (Healing system)+ 2. Spiritual Healing. I. Title.

RZ403.R45P465 2004
615.8'51—dc22   2004054100

Llewellyn Worldwide does not participate in, endorse, or have any authority or responsibility concerning private business transactions between our authors and the public.

All mail addressed to the author is forwarded but the publisher cannot, unless specifically instructed by the author, give out an address or phone number.

Any Internet references contained in this work are current at publication time, but the publisher cannot guarantee that a specific location will continue to be maintained. Please refer to the publisher's website for links to authors' websites and other sources.

Llewellyn Publications
A Division of Llewellyn Worldwide Ltd.
2143 Wooddale Drive
Woodbury, MN 55125-2989
www.llewellyn.com
Llewellyn is a registered trademark of Llewellyn Worldwide Ltd.

 Printed in the United States of America on recycled paper

Other Works by Christopher Penczak

City Magick: Urban Spells, Rituals and Shamanism

Spirit Allies: Meet Your Team from the Other Side

The Inner Temple of Witchcraft: Magick, Meditation and Psychic Development

The Inner Temple of Witchcraft CD Companion

Gay Witchcraft: Empowering the Tribe

The Outer Temple of Witchcraft: Circles, Spells and Rituals

The Outer Temple of Witchcraft CD Companion

The Witch's Shield

Sons of the Goddess: A Young Man's Guide to Wicca

The Temple of Shamanic Witchcraft: Shadows, Spirits and the Healing Journey

The Temple of Shamanic Witchcraft CD Companion

Mystic Foundation

Instant Magick

Ascension Magick: Ritual, Myth & Healing for the New Aeon

The Temple of High Witchcraft

The Temple of High Witchcraft CD Companion

The Living Temple of Witchcraft Volume One: The Descent of the Goddess

The Living Temple of Witchcraft, Volume One CD Companion

The Living Temple of Witchcraft Volume Two: The Journey of the God

The Living Temple of Witchcraft, Volume Two CD Companion

The Witch's Coin: Prosperity and Money Magick

The Witch's Heart: The Magick of Perfect Love & Perfect Trust

Acknowledgments

I thank Laura Gamache for her love, support, and introduction to Reiki. I thank Rosalie for being my first client and urging me on the path, and I thank Ronald and Steve for their love and support. I thank my Reiki Master, Joanna Pinney-Buel. Special blessings to Brenda Armstrong-Champ for inviting me to the New England Reiki Conference and planting the seed that would become this book. Thanks to Alixaendreia for her input and advice, to Leandra Walker for her last-minute rescues, and to all those who have graciously shared symbols and added to the traditions of magick and Reiki, including John Armitage, Kathleen Milner, Diane Ruth Shewmaker, Susan Isabel, Loril Moondream, Lyn Roberts-Herrick, Jamie Gallant, Derek O'Sullivan, Kat Coree, and Jessica Arsenault.

Contents

Figures

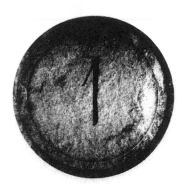

Magick and Reiki

This is not a traditional Reiki book. Although you'll find much of the basic information about what Reiki is as a healing art, including history, hand positions, and the like, you won't find a conservative view of the art of Reiki. *Magick of Reiki* is an exploration of the many systems of healing now called Reiki, viewed as a magickal tradition. Most people in the traditional Reiki community would not consider Reiki a form of magick. Most practitioners of true magick would not consider Reiki a relation to their craft. I have used both in my practice, and find them incredibly healing, valuable, and spiritual. To me, they are facets of the same force, simply using a different mechanism, and the mechanisms themselves are not that different when closely examined. As I explore both communities, there is far more crossover between the two than most believe, but no one is talking about the similarities between Reiki and magick. So now we begin a dialogue that many may find controversial. Now we bring together two worlds that have always overlapped.

Through this work, we'll explore many aspects of Reiki, and give applications of its use for the traditional Reiki practitioner as well as those involved in the magickal arts. If both topics are new to you, this book will give you a simple, firm understanding of both arts and how they relate to each other. *Magick of Reiki* is not a Reiki teaching manual for the average Reiki class, but it could be used as a manual by those teachers discussing these complementary topics along with the traditional Reiki material, or by those with a strong interest or background in metaphysics and magick. Ultimately, this book is a starting point for further discussion and experimentation.

What Is Reiki?

When I first learned Reiki, it was described to me as "universal life force" or "universal energy." That seemed pretty vague at the time, but the concept behind those lofty words is the fundamental energy that creates and sustains the universe. The *ki* in "Rei-ki" refers to the energy component. Different cultures recognize life energy and call it by different names. Ki is used in Japan. Chi is another name for basic life energy, also used in the East. The discipline of tai chi is learning how to work with this force. Hindu traditions call it prana. Hawaiian shamans call it mana. Rauch is the Hebrew term for this force. Numen, odic force, and orgone are all variant names. The different cultures have different definitions, interpretations, and cultural associations for it, but basically they are all talking about the same life energy.

This life force is found everywhere and in all things, including people, animals, and plants. It sustains us. The energy is universal, denoted by the *rei* in "Rei-ki," not personal. The universal part of the Reiki definition signifies not only that this basic energy is found in everything, universally, but also that as a system of healing, we are drawing upon this energy from the universe, which is limitless and ever abundant, rather than drawing upon our own personal "ki" or that of another person, animal, plant, or object.

Reiki the System versus Reiki the Energy

"But I already do Reiki. I didn't take any classes. I don't need to learn it from anyone." I hear this statement or something similar from many people, and it causes great debate among many in the Reiki community. The essence of the controversy comes down to a misunderstanding of terms and words. In my magickal training, I learned how important it is to say what you mean, because of the inherent power of words. Unfortunately, for most of us, English can be an imprecise language and is particularly limited when explaining mystical and Eastern concepts. Because our language often lacks the subtlety needed, we must explain things clearly.

When people say the word Reiki, some are referring to the energy of the universal life force, which is ever abundant and available to everyone. We already have some of it flowing through us every day. If we didn't, we wouldn't be alive. We take it in with the air we breathe and the food we eat, and subtly exchange it with the environment around us, including the Earth, Sun, Moon, stars, plants, and animals. There are many mystical ways to access this energy, which some people do intuitively, with little training. Many healing and magickal arts call upon this energy of the universe. Prayer, meditation, ritual, visualization, affirmations, and intent are all methods to connect to it, and they all come with their own techniques, strengths, and drawbacks. I'm sure that many people are already using this universal life force in their own way, even if they have never even heard the word Reiki.

Other people use the word Reiki to refer to a formal system of healing, originally called the Usui System of Natural Healing by its modern founder, Dr. Mikao Usui. This system has a fairly modern history, and practitioners of it have a lineage where they can trace their teachers back to Usui. The system uses specific symbols, hand positions, philosophies, and techniques, and is said to have a great many personal benefits and "safeguards" built into it. Although there are many variations and additions to it, Reiki as a system is a tradition. Without learning the tradition from a qualified teacher, you do not receive the same benefits and safeguards.

People will talk about Reiki as ancient, and the energy itself is ancient. Many people throughout history, known and unknown, have tapped into it. It is a part of life. But as a specific tradition as we know it now, Reiki is fairly modern. Perhaps its modern form is a revival of an ancient system of knowledge, as suggested by many teachers, but we have no definitive proof of this.

When people "already do Reiki" but have not studied the system nor been initiated into the tradition, they are using the energy, but are doing it in a different way than a Reiki practitioner. Sometimes that can be wonderful, and other times less so. Often there is a greater need for intense concentration, and without the safeguards, there is more of a chance that they will use too much or too little energy, or even start taking on the symptoms and illnesses of their clients, particularly if they are strictly intuitive and haven't learned a tradition of healing. Many lack the training and awareness to regulate the energy, while others do it quite beautifully on their own. It is different with each healer. But when one is a part of the tradition of Reiki, one has the ability to regulate the energy and be protected from the client's illnesses and issues.

Medical Reiki and Mystical Reiki

Medical Reiki and mystical Reiki are emerging as the two strongest schools of thought in the healing community today. Some practitioners and teachers are focusing on the medical legitimacy of Reiki in the scientific community. They participate in research projects and lobby for Reiki to be brought into the hospital and doctor's office. They teach it to healthcare practitioners, nurses, and doctors. They lobby insurance companies to cover the costs of Reiki sessions. They see it as a complementary practice to traditional and alternative medicine and seek legitimacy in the way acupuncture, Chinese medicine, Aryuveda, yoga, and some aspects of herbalism have been accepted by modern medicine. I agree that Reiki is a wonderful complement to modern medicine. It works. If it didn't, I wouldn't be using it. But some people feel the need to take out all this "mumbo jumbo" in the Reiki community and divorce it from talk about spirituality, enlightenment, spirit guides, angels, and magick. I disagree with this approach.

I can completely understand the desire to remove less mainstream ideas from Reiki when presenting it to the medical community, but Reiki as a system of healing from Japan was born out of concepts of Buddhism, a spiritual path. Although a lot of non-Buddhist philosophies have been grafted to it, the concepts behind it are essentially spiritual healing, not medical healing. For many, Reiki is not a religion, it is their spiritual path. It is the path of exploration. Reiki is a path of the mystic. And I hope in the search for legitimacy in the "straight" world that it never loses its mystical roots. *Magick of Reiki* is an effort, in light of the scientific studies now available on Reiki, to show that the foundation of many mystical traditions can be found in Reiki.

What Is Magick?

Magick is a word that evokes many reactions. For some, it evokes a sense of childhood mystery, from timeless stories and fairy tales. It conjures a belief in the endless possibilities of an innocent wish. Most think of it as make-believe or fantasy, or associate it with sleight-of-hand stage illusions. Practitioners of the spiritual art of magick use a *k* at the end to differentiate it from stage magic. I've even seen some spell it as magik or majik. But to many, the very thought of magick as a reality is a fearful prospect, drawing images of evil witches and wizards casting curses and creating harm with the wave of a hand. The remnants of magick have become our jumbled superstitions. The very concept of magick has been misunderstood for centuries by the modern culture, but it is making a resurgence in the world as we look to the ancient wisdom of the past. All ancient cultures had some form of magick as a part of their society and spiritual path.

Ultimately, magick is the power of intention. Through the use of intention, we create a change in our reality. Some magick affects our inner reality, and goes unseen by most. Other acts of magick affect the outer reality, and make things happen, although these events are most often chalked up to coincidence. You do magick to get a new job, and suddenly you get a call back for an interview and the job turns out to be perfect for you. Magick or coincidence? I was inclined to believe it was a coincidence when I started, but after repeated personal experiences involving many bizarre coincidences, I have found that there is something very real about magick. You send your intent throughout the universe, and those who can help respond to it.

Magick often takes a more ordinary approach to reach us, because that is easiest. Nature seeks to conserve energy. Water flows down mountains, not up. Magick flows down to us via the easiest path possible. We must still follow up with some real-world action. We won't get that job if we don't send our résumé and go on interviews. We must open the doors to magick. We must create that change internally, and be open to the energy, as we open to change externally. To the magickal practitioner, there is little difference between the inner reality and the outer reality. They are simply different viewpoints. To make a change in one, you must make a change in the other.

In a formal magickal tradition, practitioners focus their intention and will to create a change through the acts of ritual. Each ritual is used to create a "spell" or a specific act of magick. Rituals vary from tradition to tradition, but this type of magick is found in many different cultures.

These magickal rituals can be found in the traditions of witchcraft throughout the centuries as well as the modern revival of witchcraft and paganism. But they are also found in early forms of Jewish, Christian, and Muslim mysticism. A tradition of magick called ceremonial magick blends aspects of Judeo-Christian mysticism with philosophies from the ancient pagan civilizations, particularly Greece and Egypt. Practitioners of ceremonial magick are called magicians or mages. Rituals are also found in the shamanic cultures, among the medicine men and women of existing tribal cultures. Although they might use the word medicine instead of spell or magick, in essence they are practicing magick. A rain dance, healing song, or blessing for protection are all forms of magick.

Some spells in the form of specific acts, words, or formulas are passed on from one practitioner to another. Certain spells use very simple words and gestures, and household items. Many spells use herbs, talismans, and symbols to focus and evoke the power. They can be complicated or simple, depending on the practitioner. But the heart of magick is creating a connection to the universe, to the divine, however you envision it, and then through that connection, focusing your intention to create a change.

We all do magick all the time. We don't call it magick, but if we live with intention, any intention at all, we are doing magick. Certain forms of magick have been popularized in our modern culture and are considered somewhat respectable. Creative visualization is a form of magick. Most magickal traditions teach visualization in detail not only to help you master your mind and thoughts, but also to help you create magick.

We also call magick "the power of positive thinking." Affirmations are a form of magick. The power of our thoughts and words is a basic component of spells. Most people think that their words are powerless, but good magickal practitioners always watch what they say and think because words have power. Even if you aren't doing a formal ritual, if there is enough emotion, intent, and energy behind your thoughts or words, the universe will respond by creating a change within you. So be careful what you wish for, because you might just get it, even if you didn't really mean it.

Prayer is another form of magick. Certain people pray in a give-and-take fashion: "God, if you give me this, I will give up that." That isn't really magick, and doesn't often work. Others will ask for things, but focus so hard on their lack of what they want, or feel so unworthy to receive anything, that they don't have any energy behind their intent. Then there are those people who pray in a confident manner, feel connected to their source through unconditional love, knowing that the divine is abundant, and believe that if it is for the highest good, their prayer will be answered. And it is. They are doing magick.

Ultimately, magick is partnering with the universe to create change. Some people call it co-creating, and that's a good name. It's a blend of your will and intent, and the universe's will, or divine will. According to magickal philosophies, what you do comes back to you stronger. That is the heart of magick. It's not a moral or religious judgment, but simply a mechanism of energy. When you put out an intention, it returns to you.

Magickal power is neither good nor evil. It is simply energy. Performing magick is manipulating this energy through the power of your intention. According to the ethics of magick in its various forms, you send out only what you would want to receive, so you do no harm to others, because you would want no harm done to you. This is a variation of the Golden Rule: "Do unto others as you would have them do unto you." In witchcraft, it is called the Wiccan Rede: "An it harm none, do what ye Will." People talk about "white" magick and "black" magick, but most practitioners do not use those words. If they do, they are "dumbing it down" and explaining it in simplistic terms to those who don't want to see the complexity of intention and thought. Magick is like electricity, without moral value. It can be used to light a room or to electrocute, depending on the intent. Magick is a part of everyone and everything, like the universal life force. To me, magick is the universal life force. It is divinity in motion.

In the end, whether we are engaged in ritual, prayer, or even day-to-day action, every thought, every word, and every deed is an act of magick. Our whole life is a prayer. Our whole life is magick. Those who understand this take responsibility for their thoughts, words, and deeds because they know the power and responsibility we all have in creating reality. Everything we do affects everything else. We are all connected in the magickal web of life.

The Intersection of Reiki and Magick

Most people would assume that there is little common ground between magick and Reiki. Magick is most strongly associated with the occult and with the Western mystery traditions. The word occult simply means "hidden" and comes from the word ocular, referring to the eye. Occult subjects are those not seen, or studied, by everyone. They are obscure, and usually hidden by mystery and symbolism. Reiki comes to the world from Japan, rooted in the Eastern traditions and philosophies. On the surface, there seems to be a great division between Eastern and Western knowledge, and truly, there are many differences. But essentially they can be looked at as two different paths up the same mountain.

Magick is strongly associated with the use of magickal symbols and alphabets. Even the word spell denotes the power of the written word, when intentions are spelled out in letters and words. Magickal alphabets, symbols of power and creation, are found in many traditions. From Egyptian hieroglyphics and ancient Hebrew and Greek, to the Norse runes, Celtic ogham, and the script of the alchemists, symbols carry not only meaning, but also power inherent in their name and shape.

In Reiki, as one continues on to the second level of traditional training, the student is taught three practitioner symbols used to enhance and facilitate the practice of healing. Even though Reiki is said to be guided by the higher intelligence, and we have no control or attachment to the outcome, we do have intent when using a symbol, since we pick the symbol we are using, intuitively or logically, based on the intention behind the symbol. The first symbol is used to increase power, the second symbol is used for healing on the mental and emotional levels, and the third symbol is used for distance healing. The use of Reiki symbols in healing, by either visually drawing them or chanting their name, is like using magickal symbols and words of power.

The tradition of Reiki is passed on not only through oral or written material to be learned by the student, but most importantly through something called an attunement. Initiation is another word for attunement. The Reiki Master, or Reiki teacher, creates an energetic connection to the student, through intention and symbol, to pass on the ability to effortlessly and safely tap into the universal life force. Side effects of the attunement can be physical, mental, emotional, or spiritual cleansing and purging, awakening of intuitive or psychic abilities, and a greater awareness of spirituality and the call to higher service. This creates a spiritual family or lineage of teachers and students who are all connected and can ultimately be traced back to the modern founder of Reiki, Dr. Usui. If the teacher is not attuned already, then the connection cannot be passed on to the student. In very traditional Reiki, the sacredness of the symbols is maintained by keeping them secret from the unattuned, and the ritual of attunement is kept secret, even from lower initiates. I remember asking my Reiki Masters, after my first attunement, what exactly had happened. How did they "attune" me? They would not tell me. They didn't mention symbols or anything else. It was only thanks to my more open and modern Reiki Two teacher that I understood the mechanism of attunement.

In many magickal traditions, a key component to the experience is an awakening through initiation. Through this initiation, the teacher awakens the students to the energy the teacher holds from his or her own attunement in the tradition. Initiates report an awakening of their third eye to psychic vision and increased spiritual awareness, or a strengthening of their magickal abilities to both manifest and receive information. Many feel a stronger connection to the divine, often through a particular patron goddess or god.

Through the initiation, the student is connected to the spiritual "family" of the tradition, a magickal lineage that can be traced back to the modern founders. In the tradition of Wicca called Gardnerian Wicca, initiates can trace their lineage back to Gerald Gardner. Not only do practitioners of magickal traditions often keep their lineage a secret to the uninitiated, but the rites, symbols, and rituals of the order are also shrouded in mystery.

Initiation, awakening, spiritual lineage, symbols, energy, and secrecy are all common points in the history of magick and Reiki. Both are seen as esoteric or mystical arts that are not easily understood by the general public. Most people in the general public have no interest in these topics. Those who are seekers find the arts of magick and Reiki. Neither art is a religion in the strictest definition of the word, but both have religious aspects to them, having roots in religions. Both are mystical paths that anyone from almost any religion can practice, if they are open to the mystical path of personal experience.

Reiki and magick differ in their approach to creating change. In most traditions of magick, you form an intention and reflect upon it. You reflect to make sure that you truly desire the potential outcome. You reflect to make sure that this outcome is for the highest good, harming none. Ideally, you reflect on the effects and repercussions of magick. Then you send the energy of that specific intention out to the universe through magickal ritual. You release the intention and assume that if it is for the highest good, then the magick will work. You can follow up the magick with real-world action to open the doors to the results of your magick, but you must fully release your intention. By releasing your attachment to the result of your intention, you send the energy out to manifest the intention. If you don't release it, you will constantly pull back the energy you sent out, and it will never manifest. When the energy does return to you, as all things return to their source energetically stronger than when they left, it will return as a manifestation rather than an intention.

Reiki, on the other hand, focuses much less on outcome. The practitioner is unattached to the outcome, and simply offers Reiki energy to the recipient for his or her highest good. The recipient uses the energy to heal according to his or her own divine wisdom. Reiki is said to be regulated by the divine intelligence, the universal intelligence of this life force energy, which knows infinitely more than our conscious ego selves how to work. We simply offer ourselves as vessels through which the energy flows, and it works as needed.

Reiki energy flows where it is needed. If a practitioner's hands are on you and you need Reiki for the highest good, the energy will flow. If the practitioner is touching your chest, but you really need the energy in your toes, it will flow to your toes. If you come in for a backache, but the energy serves the highest good by going to your emotional body to help heal an unresolved childhood trauma, it will go there. There is no controlling or predicting the results of Reiki. Practitioners release attachment to the outcome. The recipient and practitioner may have a specific intention in mind before the session, and that may set the tone for the session, but there is no guarantee of the results. Reiki energy goes where commanded by one's higher intelligence in concert with the universal life force.

Magick originally evolved out of the desire to heal and meet the needs of the tribe. Traditions of hands-on healing can be found in many ancient and modern magickal and shamanic cultures. The practice was so widespread that it found its way into the teachings of Jesus and early Christianity. In Celtic traditions, people gifted with the ability to heal through touch are said to have the "faery touch" or "faery hands." Reiki's primary way of directing energy is through touch, and practitioners are known for the heat and energy that radiates from their hands.

Reiki and magick have much in common, particularly in regard to letting go. Western esoteric traditions aren't all that different from Eastern mysticism. In magick, one seeks to consciously partner with the divine. The contemplation, reflection, and intention of the "highest good" are to align with what magicians call divine will. When Wiccans and magicians say "Do what ye Will," they mean do your higher will, what the divine self wants and not necessarily what the ego wants. When the conscious mind is aligned with the divine will, magick can do anything. But there must be that alignment. If our intention is not aligned with the divine, we ask that it not come true.

In Reiki, there is not as great a need to have a specific intention. Ideally, there is no focus on the outcome. There is usually an intention, conscious or unconscious, but it's not the primary focus. In magick, the tradition involves becoming consciously aware of your desires, needs, and intentions. Both Reiki and magick are paths to awareness and openness to the divine. Both are paths of healing and wholeness. They don't need to be mutually exclusive in our lives, just as we don't have to focus strictly on left-brain or right-brain talents, or on male or female traits. We are an amalgam of both approaches to life, as found in Reiki and Western magick, and those on the balanced path will see the wisdom in both approaches.

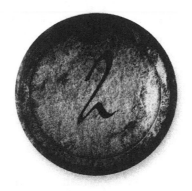

The Reiki Mythos

So now that you know more about Reiki, where does it come from? Who discovered it? It depends on if you are talking about Reiki the energy or Reiki the system. Through our exploration of the Reiki mythos, we will walk the halls of its traditional history, separating fact from less-than-fact. But in the end, as with all myths, we will discover that there are few facts that are accepted by everyone. There are many versions, many truths. We are not seeking to debunk or disprove, but instead to explore the possibilities and find which personal truths resonate with us and can be most helpful on our path. Stories can be the greatest teaching tool in explaining truth, as long as both the student and teacher remember that mythic truths are not absolute truths.

The Way I Heard It

This version of the Reiki story is very close to the first version I heard in my own First Degree Reiki training. It is passed down from teacher to student in most traditional classes. Although this version is said to be the story passed down from the three main Grandmasters of the Usui tradition of Reiki, it's interesting to notice how the story changes. I've witnessed this when talking to other Reiki Masters. It's like the gossip game. When you tell a story to someone at a party, and that person tells another, who tells another, by the end of the night, the story being told barely resembles the original story. Hopefully, in the context of a class, one would take greater care in recounting a sacred story than in relaying party gossip, but it's human nature to change, adapt, or exaggerate the facts. Since much of the Reiki tradition is considered secret and is unwritten, there are not a lot of historical written documents, and some scholars claim that the existing documentation conflicts with the story.

The founder of the modern Reiki tradition, Dr. Mikao (some say Mikaomi) Usui, was a Christian minister and a teacher at Doshisha University in Kyoto, Japan. His story begins in the late 1800s.

While teaching a class, Dr. Usui was asked by his students if he believed in the Bible literally; if he believed that Jesus could heal by laying his hands on someone. Dr. Usui answered in the affirmative, and his students asked him to prove it was possible by giving a demonstration. Dr. Usui declined, telling his students that while he believed that such things were possible, he couldn't do them. But he wanted to prove to his students that belief in such healing work was not simply blind faith. Usui quit his job at the university to study the Bible in a Christian country, the United States, studying at the University of Chicago.

While in the United States, Dr. Usui realized that the Bible wasn't taught any differently there than in Japan. No secret of healing was revealed in the English texts. He also discovered other philosophies and was attracted to Buddhism. He read accounts of Buddha healing by laying his hands on others, just like Jesus. He devoted his time to studying Buddhism, hoping to discover the secret of healing. After seven years, he returned to his hometown of Kyoto, wishing to continue his studies in a Buddhist country.

While in Japan, he spoke to many Buddhist and Zen monks, seeking knowledge. They all told him that they were only interested in spiritual healing, not in healing the physical body. He began a more in-depth study of the sutras, first in Japanese and then the Chinese version from which they were translated. Not only did Dr. Usui teach himself Chinese, he also learned Sanskrit, to better understand Buddha's original culture. In the Sanskrit documents, Usui found a formula for healing, written in special symbols, but was unsure how to use it, if it would work, and what effect it would have on the user. He decided to make a pilgrimage to request higher guidance from the divine.

After consulting with the monks, Dr. Usui decided to go on a twenty-one day retreat, fasting with only water, on Mount Koriyama, a sacred space known for granting wisdom during meditation. He told the monks to come looking for his body if he did not return by the twenty-second day.

Usui climbed the mountain, made camp, and piled twenty-one stones together. Every day he threw one stone away and spent the day meditating, praying, chanting, drinking water, and listening. Every day the same thing happened—nothing. He was expecting a revelation about how to use the formula, but got nothing.

On the twenty-first day, he began what he knew would be his last meditation. He saw a flicker of light, growing bigger and brighter, coming toward him. He opened his eyes to receive it, and almost like a lightning bolt, it struck him. He thought he was dead because he could feel nothing. Then bubbles of light surrounded him. In the bubbles he saw golden symbols of healing from the formula he had learned.

The experience was over as quickly as it began, and Usui rose, feeling wonderful. Even though he had fasted for twenty-one days, he felt vital and strong. So strong, in fact, that he felt he was able to walk down the mountain and back to Kyoto. He was not hungry or weak, and felt this was a miracle!

While climbing down the mountain, Dr. Usui stubbed his toe, ripping the nail. Blood came from his toe, and he reached down and held it instinctively until the pain disappeared. He looked down and saw his toenail back in place, completely healed. Thus he took note of his second miracle off the mountain.

As he descended, Usui came to an eating house that welcomed the monks who traditionally fasted on the mountain. The monk there was preparing the soft gruel for Usui, knowing his digestive system wouldn't be able to handle anything else after a long fast. Usui insisted on eating a traditional Japanese breakfast. The man warned him, but Usui did not heed his advice. Finally, the man gave Usui the traditional food, feeling he was not responsible for any indigestion.

The man's daughter, or perhaps granddaughter, brought out the food. A white bandage was wrapped around her head, tied in "rabbit ears." She told Usui she suffered from a toothache and couldn't get to a dentist. Usui listened to her story and placed his hands on her jaw. When he stopped, she took off the bandage, explaining that the toothache had disappeared. She got her father and said, "He is not an ordinary monk. He makes magick." Because of this miracle of magick, the father offered his gratitude to Usui and the only thing he had to offer, the food. Usui ate and digested the food with no problem, and considered the healing of the toothache and his lack of digestive pain to be the third and fourth miracles as he came off the mountain. Eventually, Usui made it back to the monks and shared both his story and Reiki with them.

Dr. Usui decided to test the power of Reiki by going to the local slums near Kyoto. The slum community was organized much like a tribe, and he was brought to the tribal leaders. They agreed to give him food and shelter in return for healing people, but Usui was forced to live like a beggar while living among beggars, giving up his money belt and trading his clothes for rags.

Usui discovered that those with long-term illnesses, having had them for longer periods of time, took longer to heal. Those who were younger, who had been ill for shorter periods of time, healed more quickly. After they were healed, Usui encouraged them to go back into society and lead productive lives, which each Reiki client did, leaving the slums behind.

After seven years of healing the sick in the poorest slums, Usui came across a familiar patient. He realized that this person was one of the first beggars he had healed. Usui was dismayed and questioned him. The answer was shocking to Usui. This man simply felt it was easier to be a beggar than to live in traditional society. Some say Usui was so upset by the greed of this person, not wanting to give back and contribute to the world, that he left the slums in sadness and anger.

Feeling he had learned from the errors of his past, Usui started his tradition of healing not only to heal others as he had done in the slums, but also to teach people how to heal themselves and others through Reiki. He would not go to them like he had gone to the beggars. Now people would seek him out and he would work with those who truly wanted to be healed. He began his practice and started the Usui System of Natural Healing.

The Way It Really Happened?

Much of this Usui mythos doesn't really ring true with some commonsense points and facts revealed later. Doesn't it seem a bit silly that Usui "discovered" the merits of Buddhism in the United States, particularly when he lived in Japan and was buried in a Buddhist temple? Perhaps he was always a Buddhist, but this Christian context was added when teaching Reiki to Christians. "If Jesus did it, then it must be okay" seems to be the message. It's also interesting to note that there is no record of Usui teaching at Doshisha University or ever attending the University of Chicago. There is no legal record of him being a doctor, either scholastically or medically. Perhaps it was an honorary title given to him later in life by his Reiki students, perhaps not. To some Reiki practitioners, even the discussion of such topics is tantamount to sacrilege, but I think it never hurts to look under all rocks and explore all possibilities.

The Myth Continues: Usui's Successors

According to the American version of the Reiki story, Dr. Chujiro Hayashi, a retired Japanese naval officer, met Dr. Usui after a lecture in about 1925 and began to study with him. Hayashi stayed with him until Usui passed on from this world in 1930, but before he left, he named Hayashi his successor, what was eventually called Grandmaster of Reiki. Hayashi continued the clinical and teaching work of Dr. Usui.

Dr. Hayashi then met Hawayo Takata, a woman born in Hawaii to two Japanese immigrants, Mr. and Mrs. Otogoro Kawamura. Her parents hoped for a life of prosperity for their daughter, whom they had named after Hawaii, but with weak physical health, she was unable to work on the Hawaiian plantations. She became a servant and then a bookkeeper to the plantation owner, and then married the plantation accountant, Saichai Takata, in 1917. After his death in 1930 from a heart attack, she raised their two daughters on her own, but with her weak health, it caused a strain. She developed asthma, nervous exhaustion, and gall bladder disease. She was later diagnosed with a tumor, and with her respiratory problems, surgery would have been dangerous, yet it was scheduled.

While preparing in the hospital, Takata heard a voice telling her that the surgery was unnecessary. She heard it again while getting onto the operating table, and finally discussed other options with her doctor. The doctor told her about Dr. Hayashi's Reiki clinic, and his own sister's experiences there as both patient and Reiki practitioner. Takata went to the Japanese Reiki clinic for four months and recovered her health. Then she decided she wanted to not only receive Reiki, but also to practice it and become a teacher. After much debate and controversy, either because Takata was considered a foreigner or too independent of a woman for the more traditional time and culture, Hayashi finally acceded to her request. She learned Reiki One and Two in Japan, and then Hayashi followed her back to Hawaii and helped her set up her own Reiki clinic, declaring her a Reiki Master in 1938. Hayashi later declared her his successor as Reiki Grand Master in 1941.

Some say that after World War II until 1970, Takata was the only living Reiki Master in the world. Hayashi had supposedly committed suicide to prevent Reiki from getting into the "wrong" hands by the Axis powers. He had been drafted back into the military, and had sworn not to take a life. Reportedly, Hayashi willed his own heart to stop on May 10, 1941.

Strange, I thought Reiki was only for healing. So how could it be used for the wrong purposes? That's a very Western attitude. The suicide of the Japanese Reiki Masters was proven false. Reiki traditions in Japan have survived and made their presence known in the West, and they do not acknowledge Hayashi or Takata as their Grand Masters. Both Hayashi and Takata are said to have taught Reiki exactly as Usui taught it, but others claim that Hayashi added the levels, attunements, and specific hand positions.

Regardless, Takata started attuning friends and family for free, against Hayashi's explicit instructions, and found, like Usui, that people kept returning to her, never taking responsibility for their own healing nor sharing Reiki with others. She felt that not a single person had improved their own health or success after receiving their Reiki attunements, so she decided that there must be an energy exchange, often a financial one, to make sure the students understood, valued, and committed themselves to Reiki. At that time, Takata set up the controversial fee system found in many traditional Reiki systems. Some charge as much as ten thousand dollars for the Reiki Master attunement and training.

Between 1970 and 1980, Takata trained at least twenty-two Reiki Masters, who spread the teaching of Reiki to the continental United States, Europe, and Australia. Since then Reiki has spread throughout the world. Takata passed from this world on December 11, 1980. Since then, many traditions of Reiki have developed and branched off from the strict Usui system.

The Moral of the Story

The Reiki myth is most importantly a teaching tool to convey the importance of two precepts found in the tradition. In the end, the historical facts seem less important than the moral of the story.

First, the recipients of Reiki energy must ask to be healed. They must be open and willing to change, and ready to receive the healing energy. If the recipients don't want to be healed, then they will not change the patterns of illness that are holding them back in imbalance and illness. A Reiki practitioner must not try to force healing on those who don't really want to heal. So, to be sure, the recipients must seek healing or ask to receive it.

Second, an energy exchange must occur between the practitioner and the recipient. Although the energy is universal and belongs to no one individual, the practitioner must be honored for his or her time and services. Both Usui and Takata discovered that without such an exchange, others might not value it. Some practitioners see it as an "unpaid obligation." To many people, it opens up a whole can of worms regarding spirituality and money. In the end, each practitioner has to decide what works best in his or her life when it comes to exchange.

Exchanges don't have to be monetary. They can be exchanges of services and time. Family members make such exchanges all the time. I know that when I was training for Reiki, I needed a certain amount of "case studies" to complete my teacher's requirements. Friends and family gave me their time so that I could have my case studies. I continue to share Reiki with those in my personal life. But when I'm doing Reiki in the context of professional services, I usually charge, because money is the easiest system of exchange in our current society. I sometimes do things on barter, but that doesn't always pay my bills. I've had to pay for classes, a massage table, office space, advertising materials, and such to do this work, so I have to receive something to be able to continue my work. I love doing jewelry and crystal exchanges, but the bank will not accept them as payment when I need to pay my mortgage. At times I've accepted webpage design, massage therapy, personal fitness training, editing, and artwork as an exchange, since I wanted these services and would have had to pay for them myself anyway. So many times, money never has to change hands and you can still have an exchange.

Now Here's What Really Happened

The Reiki story doesn't stop there. Special practitioners with secret knowledge have revealed the true roots of Reiki. Jesus of Nazareth went to India, some say before his crucifixion, others say after his resurrection. In India, he hid the secret to his healing method so it would not be lost and could be revealed to the world when it was needed again in the last days. Jesus had received it from the ancient Egyptian priesthood when he was initiated into it as a child. The Egyptians learned Reiki from those who escaped the sinking of the continent of Atlantis. The Atlanteans were in contact with alien races, who gave the Reiki system to the ruling class of Atlantis. And in fact, Dr. Usui was abducted by aliens while on his mountain fast, and the lights he saw were the spaceships imparting their energy technology to him. And that's what really happened!

Don't you believe me? I've heard bits and pieces of all these tales, not necessarily all tied together like that, from Reiki Masters, taught as fact. They could be facts. I believe in the ancient wisdom of India and Egypt. I believe in the possibility of Atlantis. Heck, I even believe in aliens. But I'm not sure how any of them figure into the Reiki story. They are truly possibilities, like anything else is a possibility when exploring the unknown origins of some ancient Reiki system, if indeed there was an ancient Reiki system. But these bits of "history" have not been documented or proven in any real way. Any system of healing from Egypt, India, Atlantis, Jesus, or alien visitors is not the system of healing known as Reiki in the modern world.

Again, we need to make the distinction between Reiki the energy and Reiki the system. I'm sure that if a man named Jesus did healing, he was using some form of universal energy. I think the magickal traditions of India, Egypt, and any other magickal cultures use a form of universal energy. But it is not the system of healing called Reiki as we know it today. Everyone is trying to find the "ancient source" of wisdom so that Reiki will seem more mystical, magickal, and authentic. Well, the energy is ancient, but this system is modern, and there is nothing wrong with that. Reiki is a system to help modern people, and hopefully it will continue to adapt and grow as people change. Ancient isn't always better. I prefer modern plumbing to ancient plumbing. We must use what fits our society.

So many teachers take inspired material from channeling or personal belief and state it as fact, though it can't be proved. If it is presented as possibility, there is no harm, but some Reiki students know nothing about Dr. Usui and his lineage, but can tell you all about Atlantis. That's not Reiki. Certain teachers do this because that is where their interest lies, or they do it to demonstrate some superior knowledge to "regular" Reiki teachers. Many were taught it as fact, and pass it on that way, not knowing any better.

The Reiki "story" happened less than 150 years ago, yet the facts on which it is based are still fuzzy. The story has gone from factual account to mythic fiction so quickly that

I'm now starting to doubt many other "facts" in traditional history. Myths can take on a life of their own. So, while we still have time, I think it is important to preserve the more down-to-earth story of Reiki and simply leave other possibilities open. By keeping the modern myth and the ancient possibilities distinct, I think that Reiki teachers will be doing a greater service to their students and the Reiki community.

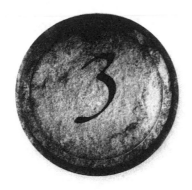

The First Degree: Reiki One

In the various traditions of Reiki, material is basically divided into several levels of study. Perhaps in Dr. Usui's day there was a longer time of apprenticeship, but in the realm of weekend workshops and spiritual intensives of the twenty-first century, Reiki has been divided into smaller packets of information and experiences that a student can process. Most teach in small groups. Some do larger lectures, and it is now very popular to teach Reiki in a one-on-one setting.

Although different teachers, particularly in the independent traditions, divide the information in the levels differently, there is a typical format that most follow. The first step in the study of Reiki, level one, is the foundation of the training. It is usually taught in a full day or even up to two days. In the class, students are taught the basic definition of Reiki and are often given a demonstration if they have had no prior experience with it. Then the Reiki myth is taught to discuss the two precepts stressed in the story: permission and exchange.

The Reiki Principles

In Reiki One, students are introduced to the basic philosophy of Reiki through what are now known as the Reiki principles. They are usually credited to Dr. Usui, but as a code of honor, they more likely originated from the Meiji Emperor of Japan. Usui passed these concepts on to his students, and in various forms they made their way through Takata to the Western Reiki student.

There are several forms of the Reiki principles, but this is the version I was taught:

Just for today, I will be grateful.

Just for today, I will not anger.

Just for today, I will not worry.

Just for today, I will do my work honestly.

Just for today, I will respect all life.

The most important part for me is the "Just for today," because it always reminds me to be in the moment. I can't control the past, I can't control the future, but I can be in the moment and remind myself of these five principles in the moment. One of the key concepts in Reiki is detachment from the outcome. When we are detached, we learn to be in the moment. We can acknowledge situations that cause anger or worry, but learn not to identify with them so closely.

Reiki teachers disagree about the importance of these principles in teaching. Since Reiki is not a religion, many feel they have their own moral code to follow. Other Reiki teachers believe that the Reiki principles are the guiding force behind the tradition of Reiki, as the founder, Dr. Usui, presented it. They can be used as daily affirmations. My friend Lisa Davenport, a well-respected Reiki teacher, really feels that these principles are the foundation of Reiki philosophy and emphasizes them in all her classes, particularly her Reiki Master classes. I tend to emphasize them less, but most of my students are witches and mages who already have their own philosophical codes to guide their lives. I teach the principles in a historical context, but don't require my students to use them as daily affirmations. I use the Reiki principles to challenge my students. By reflecting on them and discussing them, the students have to think about what moral and spiritual codes, or lack thereof, they are already using in their lives.

The Roots of Dis-Ease

A main teaching of the First Degree is the concept of spiritual and energetic healing. When I took my first Reiki class, the majority of students were from the mainstream and medical communities, not the mystical. The concept of energy healing was new to most of those attending. My first teachers, like most Reiki teachers, were challenged to convey sophisticated spiritual concepts of health in an easy-to-understand way.

Health is not just a physical phenomenon. We do not just have physical bodies. In the spiritual model of healing, we have more than one body. We have what are called subtle energy bodies. They are named in many ways, but a simple model has four bodies: physical, emotional, mental, and spiritual. When we have an illness or injury, an imbalance occurs first in our energy body before anything happens in our physical body. Disease is really "dis-ease," a lack of ease and comfort in the mind, emotions, spirit, or body. When we tense and contract our consciousness, due to fear, pain, anger, or other unresolved feelings and thoughts, we contract our energy body. If the contraction holds, energy that regulates our health cannot flow freely as needed. The block can then manifest as an illness. The spiritual block precipitates down to the more dense levels of the physical world, creating the illness.

Reiki works by gently releasing the blocks. The energy flows into the system to dislodge the blocks. Reiki goes where it serves the highest good. Although we may come in for a session to heal a pain or ache, thinking that the problem is physical, Reiki energy will flow to the root of the pain, which may lie in the emotional or mental body. Once the energetic root of the problem is healed, the physical symptoms will clear up. But during or after the session, the recipient might have to process the feelings and thoughts of the block. Sometimes processing occurs on the conscious level, and other times on the unconscious level.

My favorite symbol for the Reiki healing process is a glass of water. The recipient is like a glass of water with mud at the bottom. The mud is the blocked energy and illness. Reiki is like a stream of pure, clean water being poured into the glass. The water may agitate the mud, causing the glass of water to become cloudy. That is the processing and clearing of the energy. Eventually, the pure water flushes out the mud and sand, leaving a clear glass of healthy, pure water. We may clear one layer of mud that is ready to leave, but other layers of mud may be more resistant. They will only clear when they are ready to clear. Reiki flushes them out in a gentle, flowing way. The water doesn't know how or when the mud will clear, but simply allows the flow, and lets the process occur. The fresh, clear water pouring down can't suck up the mud and infect the source. The Reiki energy flows in a one-way direction, into the recipient, and the mud is flushed down to the earth, where it can be used again in a new form. In other words, the practitioner can't take on the unhealthy energies of the recipient. The built-in safeguards of the process don't allow this to happen. Energy cannot be created or destroyed; it can only be transmuted to a more helpful form or brought to a more suitable environment. Energy that is too dense to carry in your physical body may be useful somewhere else; just like mud does us no good in our drinking water, but can benefit our garden, once it changes back into soil.

What a great, simple image this is to convey to others about the Reiki process. The process of spiritual healing can be more complicated than this, but I think simple is the best starting place when doing healing work. Ultimately, every illness has an energetic root to it, a dis-ease that can result in health problems. Reiki, as an energy medicine, heals the root of illness, allowing the body to heal itself because the blocks to healing are cleared.

The Chakras

Reiki Masters in the West usually touch upon the chakras in the First Degree. In my Reiki One training, I was given an overview of the concept of the chakras, with no practical information. The Hindu word chakra is generally translated as "spinning wheel," referring to spinning vortexes of energy found in the human body. In reality, chakras are part of Hindu metaphysics, not Japanese, and are not part of the original Reiki system. But since so many in the "New Age" world are familiar with chakras and then take Reiki classes, the two are complementary. Personally, I find the model of the chakras to be a very helpful system of knowledge when doing healing work on myself and with others.

Each chakra energy center represents a level of consciousness in human life. Energy blocks in the body are often centered at, or connected to, a chakra point. The chakras are also associated with specific parts of the body. When we have physical illness or injury, or sense a block in a particular chakra through intuitive means, we know what level of consciousness, what issues, are at play in the healing work.

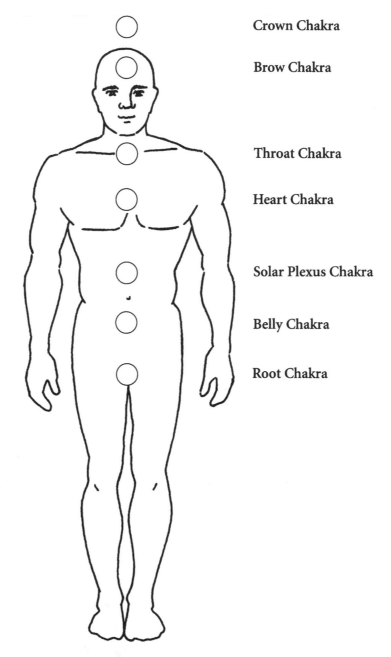

Crown Chakra

Brow Chakra

Throat Chakra

Heart Chakra

Solar Plexus Chakra

Belly Chakra

Root Chakra

Figure 1: The Seven Chakras

Root

The root chakra is usually visualized as a red disk of light at the base of the spine, or at the perineum point, between the sex organs and the anus. The root consciousness is the level of physical survival and physical pleasure, giving us the ability to be in the world. Here we have our survival instincts, sense of tribe or family, and ability to take care of our body. We see sexuality as pleasure as well as the instinct of passing on the genetic code. The root chakra is tied to the eliminative system, which eliminates toxins from the body and allows us to survive in the world. It is also tied to the reproductive system. Imbalances of the root chakra may manifest as illness in those systems, as well as feelings of not wanting to be in the world, suicidal impulses, ungroundedness, and an inability to accept pleasure from the body or senses.

Belly

The belly chakra is visualized as a ball of orange light at the navel or right below it. This center corresponds with our ability to feel and connect with others outside ourselves. We have our instincts here, gut instincts, as to whom to trust and whom not to trust. The belly chakra, also called the sacral or navel chakra, is tied to sexuality in terms of relationships, intimacy, sharing, and trust. Nourishment is also associated with this chakra since it is connected to the intestines, spleen, and lower digestive system, and it is here that we absorb food. Here we nourish ourselves, physically and emotionally. Upsets in these areas of life are signs of belly chakra imbalances.

Solar Plexus

The solar plexus chakra is a yellow or golden orb located right below the diaphragm muscle and above the navel. This is our center of power and fire. Here we work on issues of personal power and control. If we struggle with it, or let others control or sap our power, we lose energy from this space. When we are not in our true authentic power, we struggle with anger and fear. The solar plexus chakra is also tied to self-image and self-esteem. The liver, gall bladder, adrenals, and stomach are all associated with this chakra. The adrenal glands are associated with the fight-or-flight response. As the physical liver stores toxins, the energy of the liver is said to store emotional toxins such as fear, anger, and shame. Healing the solar plexus chakra heals those issues and parts of the body.

Heart

The heart chakra is the bridge between the upper and lower chakras, using the realm of emotion to connect the lower, more physical chakras with the upper, more mental and spiritual centers. It is usually visualized as a green wheel of light at the sternum, though some traditions teach that the heart chakra has a pink or red center. Here we feel not only romantic love and love for our family, but also self-love and divine, unconditional love. When we are open to love, our heart chakra feels open and free. When we lack the love vibration, we feel closed or heavy in the heart. This chakra center physically interacts with the heart muscle, circulatory system, thymus gland, and immune system. When we are not connected to love, circulatory and immune problems can arise.

Throat

At the throat center we express ourselves, our needs and our will. Here we communicate, not only by speaking, but also by listening. To truly communicate, we must be able to receive information as well as send it out. The throat chakra rules the vocal mechanisms, as well as the mouth, gums, teeth, and ears. It is visualized as blue and corresponds with the mind. Like the sky, our mind and throat chakra can be clear and bright, or clouded and heavy. When we speak our truth, the throat is clear. When we are not expressing our authentic self, vocal problems arise, including sore throats, colds, and infections.

Brow

The brow chakra is called the third eye, because at this chakra center we see with our inner vision as well as our outer vision. It is connected to the pineal gland, which senses light using mechanisms that are similar to what our eyes use to see light. Even though it exists within our brain, the third eye sees with spiritual light. Through this indigo/purple energy, we take in information psychically or intuitively, and we send out visions of our manifestations, through visualization and intention. When we don't trust our intuition or don't want to see what is around us, this chakra center closes down, resulting in either psychic blindness or physical eye problems.

Crown

The crown chakra is visualized as a sphere of dazzling white or violet light at the top of the head where the skull bones meet. It is the chakra of spiritual survival and connection, "crowning" the other six chakras in much the same way that its gland, the pituitary, regulates all other glands. The brain is the body center, and it controls the rest of the body as well. Through the crown chakra, we have a connection to the divine and to our sense of purpose in the world. Through this chakra we know and fulfill divine will, or the highest good. When the crown center is closed down, we feel disconnected and unloved by the divine, and we question the meaning of existence. Issues involving the physical nervous system, as well as any ailments that are system-wide or force a reevaluation of life roles and meaning, are crown chakra issues.

Extended Chakras

Some healers in the modern metaphysical realm use interpretations of the chakra system that include additional chakra points. Even though these new systems have many similarities, explorers into this realm often disagree about the names, locations, colors, and meanings of the additional chakras. It is possible that these chakras have been ever present in the human body throughout history. Another possibility is that a "new" range of energies may be slowly coming "online" as we enter the New Age and evolve in consciousness, which would explain why the ancients made little mention of them in the Sanskrit texts.

Though I have used this version of the chakra system in my own meditations and personal work, I have found it to be too complex to use with clients who are new to energy healing and metaphysics. At times, the concepts of chakras and energy healing can be hard enough to explain without delving into an "advanced" chakra system.

The following model locates additional chakras between the seven major chakra points, much as how the five black keys of a piano are positioned between the seven white keys in each octave. It also locates chakras above and below the normal range of seven.

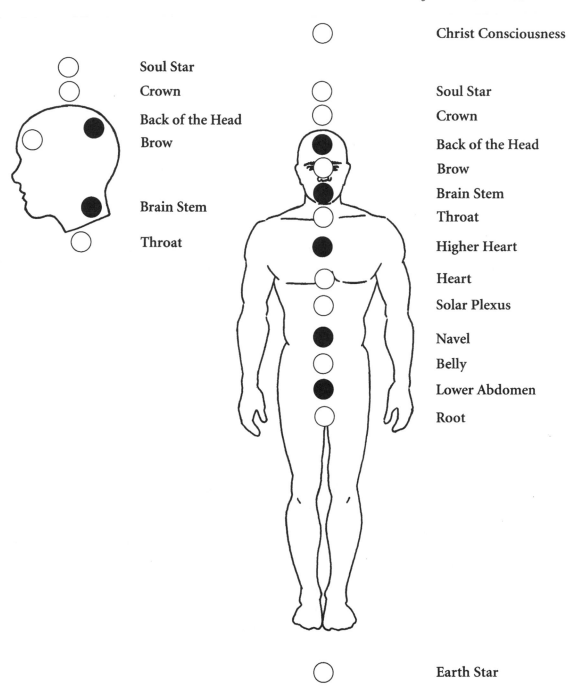

Christ Consciousness

Soul Star

Crown

Back of the Head

Brow

Brain Stem

Throat

Higher Heart

Heart

Solar Plexus

Navel

Belly

Lower Abdomen

Root

Soul Star

Crown

Back of the Head

Brow

Brain Stem

Throat

Earth Star

Figure 2: Extended Chakras

Earth Star

Earth Star is the chakra located one hand-length beneath the feet, and is visualized as black, brown, or other earth tones. It is our true connection to the planet and the physical realm. Teachers of energy evolution consider it the "crown" center of humanity's last energetic evolution, feeling that a previous chakra system descended down into the Earth, making room for our current chakra system to come into the body. Such theorists believe that the current rainbow model of chakras will eventually descend into the Earth, and then unknown chakras above the head will descend into the body as we make the next leap in consciousness.

Lower Abdomen

This red-orange center is located below the second orange belly chakra, bridging the connection between the root and belly chakras. Related to the Ovarian/Sperm Palace of Eastern traditions, it forms a link between the sexuality of the two major centers of the root and belly.

Navel

The navel chakra is pictured as yellow-orange or gold in color, and is located between the traditional orange belly chakra and the yellow solar plexus chakra. It is involved in the digestive process, and its function is learning self-control and discipline.

Higher Heart

In this model, the thymus is given its own chakra center, separate from the heart chakra and below the throat chakra. While the sternum is the center of emotion, the thymus is the place of unconditional love. The higher heart chakra is pictured as blue-green, turquoise, or aqua.

Brain Stem

The chakra center located at the base of the head can be called the well of dreams, jade pillow, or cranial pump center. Colored a deep blue, this point embodies our unconscious mind and dreams. The function of the brain stem chakra is to bring these areas into greater awareness.

Back of the Head

Visualized as magenta or violet in color, this chakra is the last point before the expansion of the crown chakra. It is the place of sacred geometry and of relating personal vision to the divine will, bridging the functions of the brow and crown chakras. Through it we move past any of our personal limits that prevent us from reaching the expanded consciousness represented by the crown chakra.

Soul Star

This chakra center is located above the crown chakra, usually several inches to several feet above it. The soul star chakra, or transpersonal point, represents the foundation of the next evolutionary leap in consciousness. It is like the "root" of our next evolution and is usually pictured in dazzling white, if with any color at all. Through it we connect to higher consciousness and the sky realms.

Christ Consciousness

This chakra is conceptualized as being above the Earth, in the lunar orbit, sometimes giving it the name of the moonstar chakra. Others conceptualize it as going into the Sun itself, since this level of consciousness is often associated with solar light and Sun gods. This chakra connects humanity to the "Christ consciousness," a relatively modern name for the awareness of all things through unconditional love.

Other chakras are conceptualized as being near the Sun, or through the Sun and into the galactic center. These chakra points are not often used in diagnosis with clients, but can be fun to conjecture about and explore in meditation. We are also said to have chakras at the major points of connection in the body, including the hands, feet, fingers and toes, elbows, knees, wrists, ankles, shoulders, and nose.

Spiritual Anatomy

Teachers who focus on the medical aspects of Reiki often spend much less time on the chakras, and may focus instead on the physical anatomy of the body. The physical body speaks to us through a symbol system that is not as esoteric as the chakra system. Each part of the body represents specific psycho-spiritual issues. Illness or injury in a particular part of the body represents a mental, emotional, or spiritual imbalance in the area of consciousness represented by that part of the body. Use this list to learn and understand the system of body symbolism.

Left Side	Feminine, receiving, personal, home, private
Right Side	Masculine, giving, projecting, work, public
Head/Face	Identity
Eyes	Seeing the world clearly, looking at the past/present/future
Ears	Listening to others, listening to the inner voice
Mouth/Teeth	Nourishment, communication
Throat	Speaking truth, communication, listening/speaking balance
Shoulder/Arm	Communication, self-expression
Hands	Dominant hand: ability to give; nondominant hand: ability to receive
Heart	Love, self-love, relationships
Bones	Support, strength, foundation, reliability
Back	Support, strength, standing in your truth, being yourself
Breast	Feminine, mother, nourishment, childhood
Stomach	Nourishment, mother
Liver	Anger, fear, resentment, feeling unprotected
Intestines	Discrimination/discernment, work, nervousness, release
Kidneys	Balance, relationships, cleansing
Reproductive	Sexuality, pleasure, family, shame
Bladder	Anger, fear
Eliminative	Fear of death, holding on to harmful energies, release
Hips	Intimacy
Thighs	Freedom, activity, action, sport, recreation
Knees/Shins	Responsibility, pressure, tension, stress, honor
Ankles	Individuality, social support, friendship
Feet	Creativity, music, art, dance, support, foundation, depression, escape

I've also found the study of medical astrology to be very helpful in finding the spiritual root of physical ailments. This discipline relates parts of the body to various signs and organs, and then correlates the spiritual issues related to each sign and planet to the illness. Chakras, symbolism, and astrology are all methods for understanding the relationship between consciousness and physical health.

The Attunement Cleanse

The first attunement to Reiki is the most critical aspect of training. Once you have received your first attunement, you can begin the practice of Reiki. In the attunement process, the Reiki Master already holds a connection to the universal life force through the symbols of the Reiki system, as passed from his or her own teacher. The attunement is a ritual, an initiation, where the teacher passes this connection on to the new student through symbols and intent. Although there are several attunements in the training, all you really need is the first one. Once you are attuned, you are connected to the universal life force through the system of Reiki, with all its inherent safeguards, for the rest of your life. Your ability to channel Reiki will develop the more you use it.

As you clear yourself as a channel, your ability to let the energy flow through you increases. My friend Erik related to me a Native American healer's words which seem to describe the Reiki philosophy perfectly: "I pray to be a hollow clean bone. The divine can then flow through me." Some describe it as a flute, to be played by God. Whatever image you use, this fits Reiki exactly. When a healer uses Reiki, he or she is also nourished and healed by it. The attunement process, and subsequent uses of the energy, initiates a healing cleanse that helps the recipient of the attunement release all unwanted forces on the physical, emotional, and mental levels.

Reiki teachers say that after each attunement, you will classically go through a twenty-one-day cleansing period. This time amount is probably an homage to Dr. Usui's experience, more than anything else. A friend of mine said it was a cleansing period for each of the seven chakras, or energy centers, of the body. One system of belief has a cleanse lasting one day for each of the chakras, starting at the root chakra and cycling through all seven chakras in three periods. Another system has each chakra and its core issues cleanse for three days, until the crown chakra is reached.

In Reiki One, the cleanse is usually characterized as being more physical. Students often have a cold, the flu, or allergy-like symptoms as their bodies purge unwanted elements. The physical aspect of Reiki is stressed at this level, focusing on hands-on healing and in-person treatments. In Reiki Two, the nature of the cleanse is usually more emotional or mental, bringing up issues of a personal nature that need to be addressed for further clarity. Level three references a more spiritual or transpersonal cleansing. These categories are only the most common experiences and not a hard-and-fast rule. Students can have a great spiritual awakening after a Reiki One attunement.

To facilitate the cleansing process, drink a lot of water during class, after class, and for the entire twenty-one-day period. Take care of yourself, getting as much rest, nutrition, and exercise as your body and soul need.

Personally, I've experienced some of these cleansing periods for a much shorter time than twenty-one days, and then later, for much longer periods, so twenty-one is only a guideline. A period of self-healing through Reiki self-treatments for twenty-one days straight is a common practice, letting you commit to the energy and to the process. I wish my Reiki One teachers had suggested it to me. But I can still do Reiki, even without that purposeful period of commitment. You don't "lose" your connection to Reiki if you don't do it for twenty-one days in a row.

Hands On = Reiki On

The most important thing you will learn in Reiki One, regardless of the cleanse or lack thereof that you experience, is that once you have been attuned, if your hands are placed on someone, including yourself, then your Reiki channel is "on." "Hands on, Reiki on," as teachers say. If the person you are touching is in need of energy, the energy will flow. You are not in control of it. The higher intelligence of the universal life force is in charge. Medical Reiki practitioners say it is the cells of the recipient's body that control how much energy is absorbed. Metaphysicians believe it is the recipient's higher self, or the recipient's own spirit guides, that are in charge of the flow of energy.

In either case, the process can be likened to sucking liquid through a straw. The practitioner is the straw, and the energy is the liquid. The recipient is "sucking" Reiki energy through a straw. The recipient controls the process on some level, and stops sucking when he or she is full and can process no more. It is not possible to overdose on Reiki energy, although your patients may undergo their own spiritual cleanse and feel like they have overdosed on it. Ultimately, regardless of the outcome, the end result is for the highest good and out of your hands.

Because you don't control the energy, if it flows, you may take that as implicit permission to give Reiki. Proper etiquette suggests, from Dr. Usui's story, that one ask outright for permission to practice Reiki, and I usually do. If someone is coming to my office for a treatment, permission is implied. But if I am counseling someone, formally or informally, and I feel the energy turn on with a familiar buzzing in my hands, then I know it is flowing for the highest good and I should let it flow. Oftentimes it would be inopportune or inappropriate for me to stop and ask outright for permission to do Reiki. I know I have the universe's permission, and that's the most important thing to me.

Once, when counseling a woman in the hospital before her husband passed on, we spoke together in the cafeteria. I had my hand on hers, and the Reiki flowed into her. She was not in a place to hear about energy or healing. She needed to talk. Later, she took Reiki classes with me, and it dawned on her what I had been doing that day. It was so simple, and she hadn't even consciously felt it at the time, but now she understands how Reiki had calmed her down. She had chalked it up to my personality, but now knows it had much more to do with the Reiki healing.

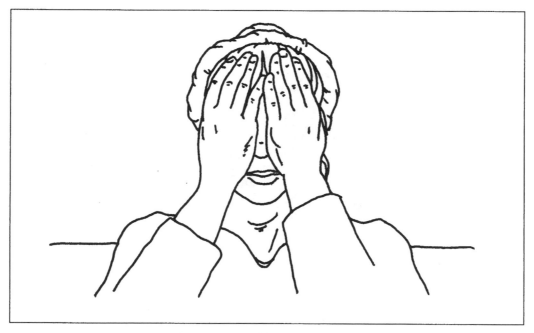

Position 1

Figure 3: Hand Positions for Self-Treatment

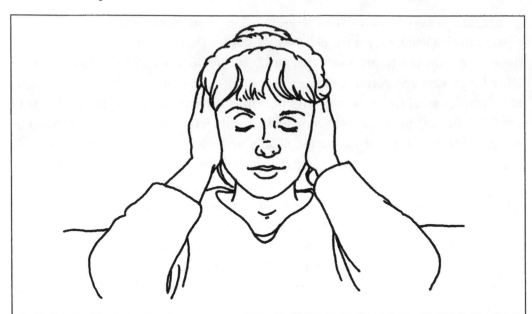

Position 2

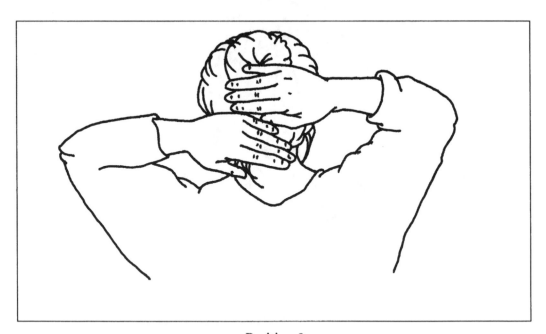

Position 3

Figure 3: Hand Positions for Self-Treatment (continued)

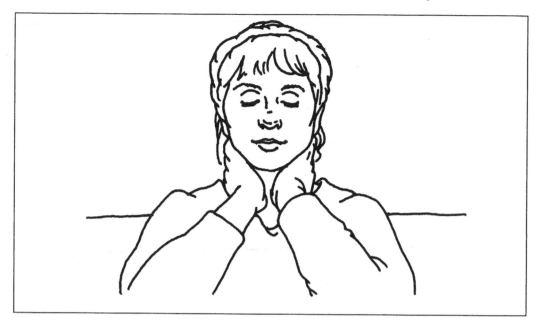

Position 4

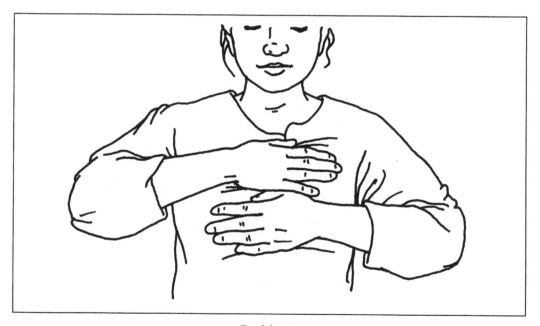

Position 5

Figure 3: Hand Positions for Self-Treatment (continued)

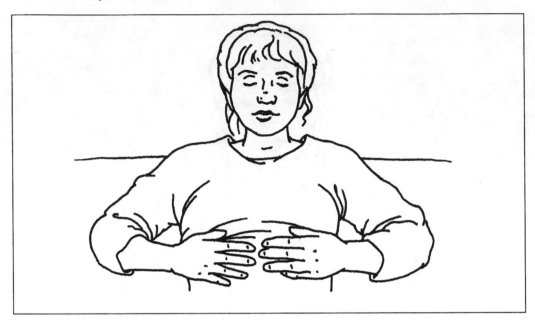

Position 6

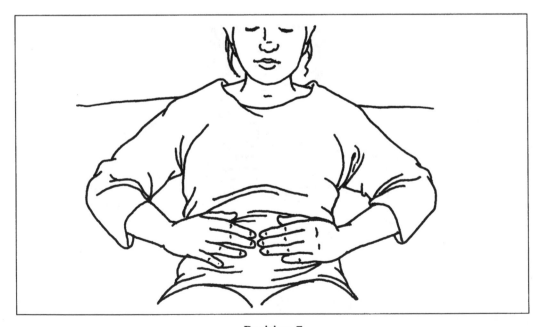

Position 7

Figure 3: Hand Positions for Self-Treatment (continued)

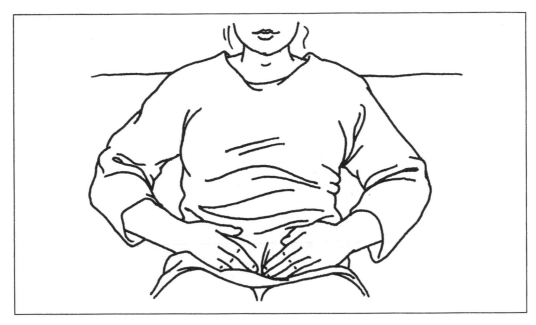

Position 8

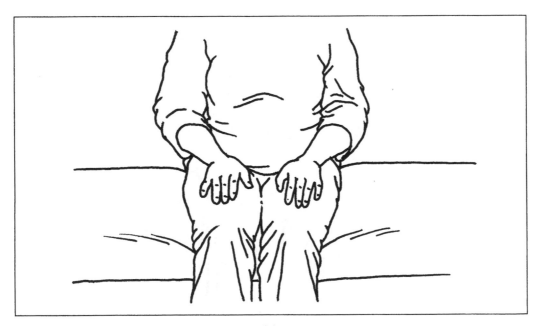

Position 9

Figure 3: Hand Positions for Self-Treatment (continued)

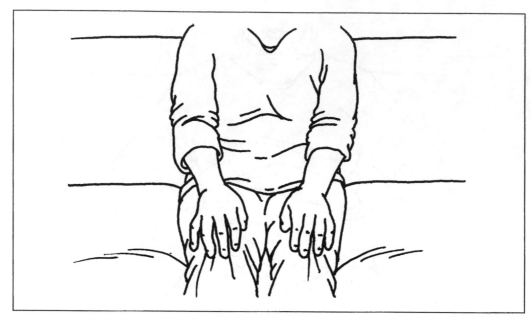

Position 10

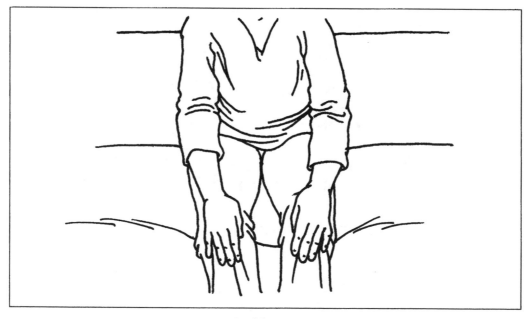

Position 11

Figure 3: Hand Positions for Self-Treatment (continued)

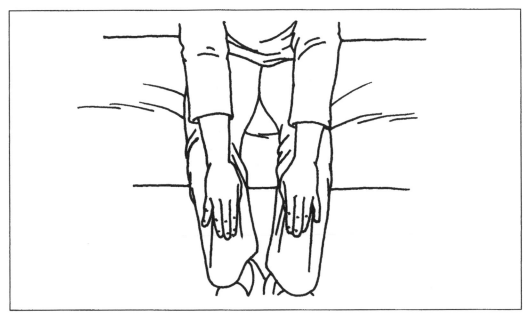

Position 12

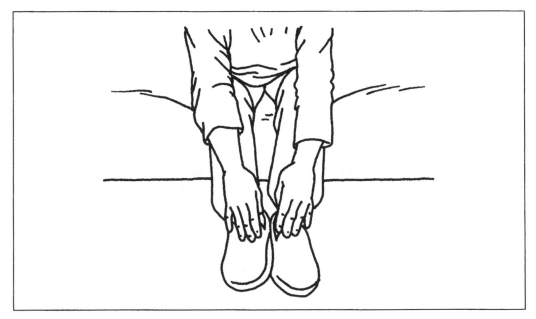

Position 13

Figure 3: Hand Positions for Self-Treatment (continued)

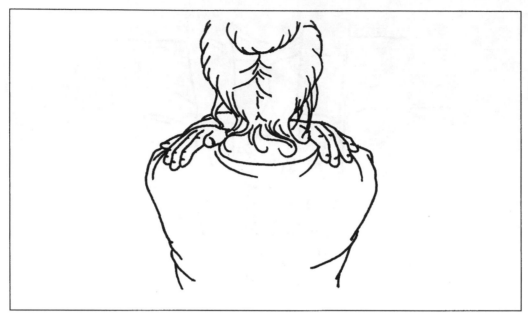

Position 14 (optional)

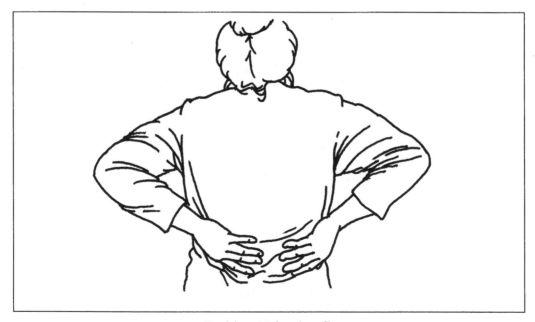

Position 15 (optional)

Figure 3: Hand Positions for Self-Treatment (continued)

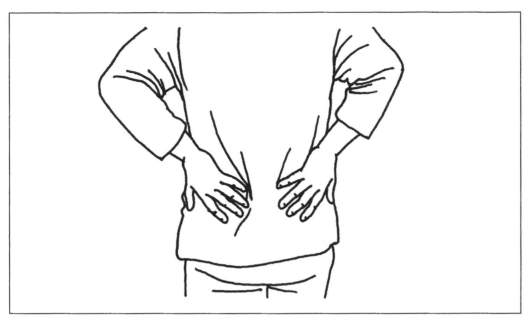

Position 16 (optional)

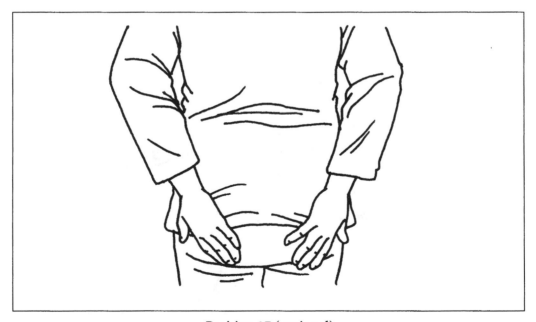

Position 17 (optional)

Figure 3: Hand Positions for Self-Treatment (continued)

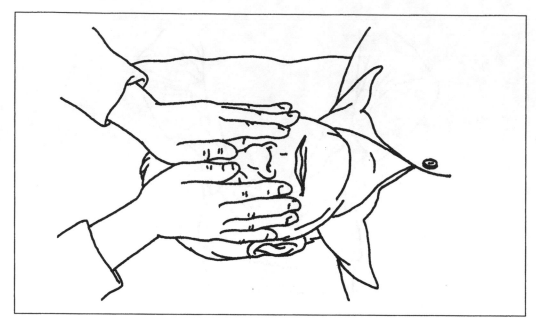

Position 1

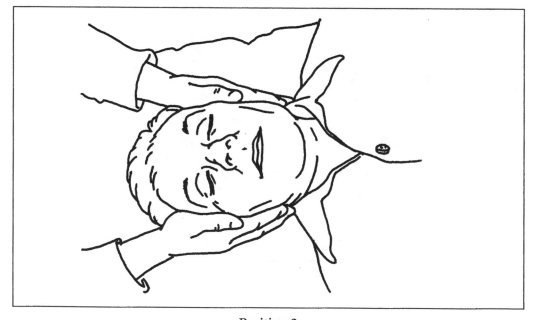

Position 2

Figure 4: Hand Positions for Treatment of Others

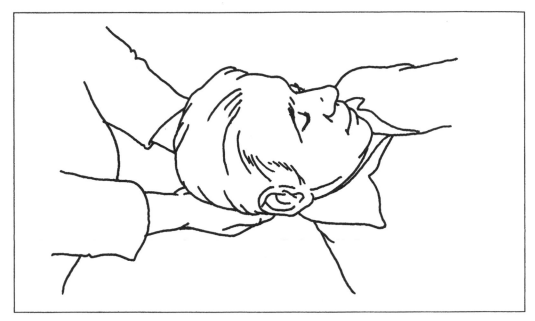

Position 3

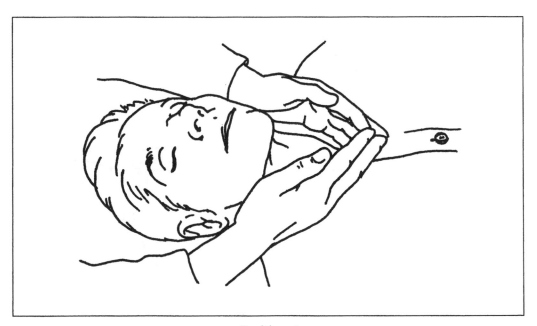

Position 4

Figure 4: Hand Positions for Treatment of Others (continued)

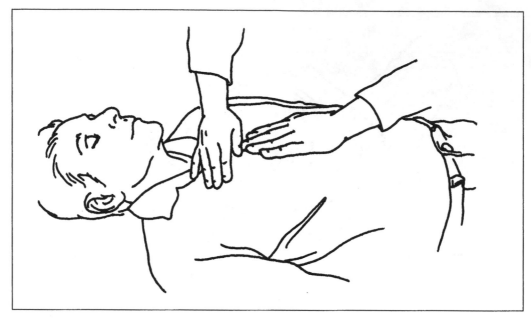

Position 5

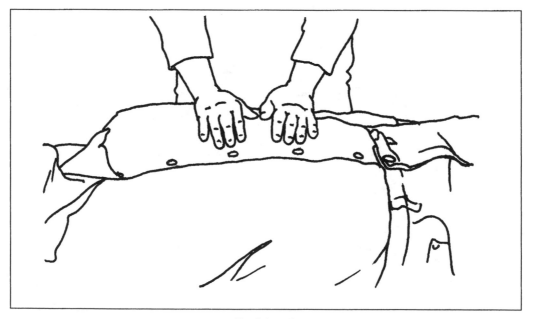

Position 6

Figure 4: Hand Positions for Treatment of Others (continued)

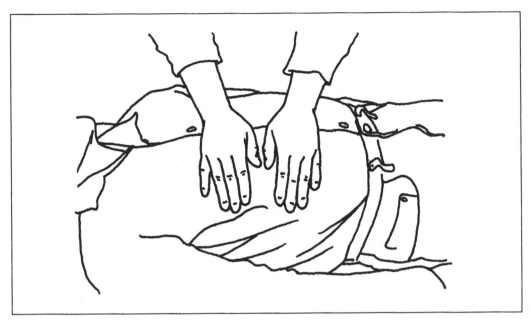

Position 7

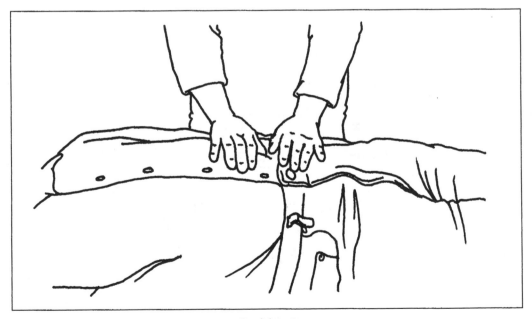

Position 8

Figure 4: Hand Positions for Treatment of Others (continued)

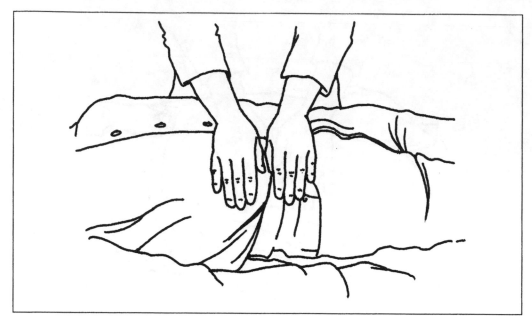

Position 9

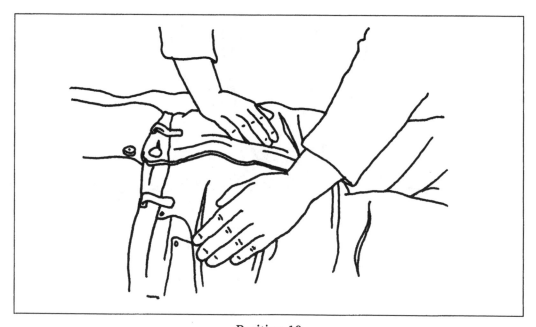

Position 10

Figure 4: Hand Positions for Treatment of Others (continued)

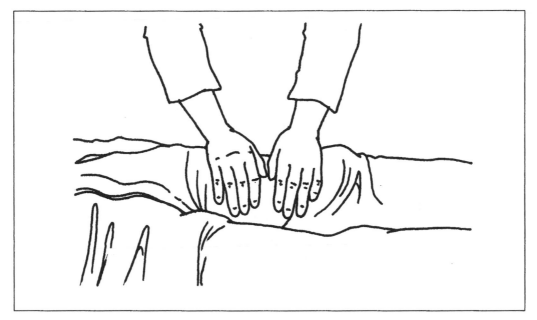

Position 11

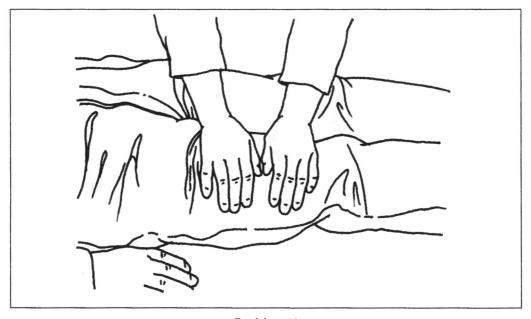

Position 12

Figure 4: Hand Positions for Treatment of Others (continued)

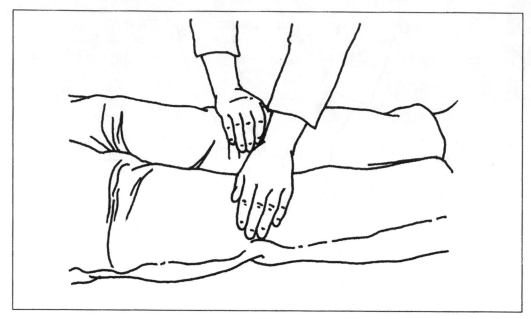

Position 13

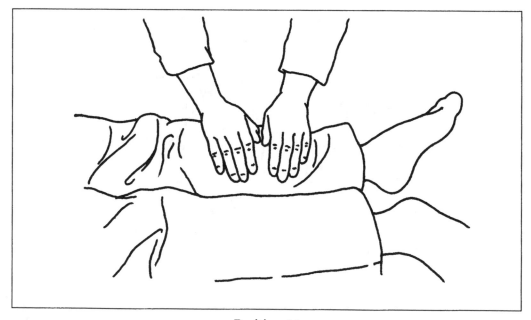

Position 14

Figure 4: Hand Positions for Treatment of Others (continued)

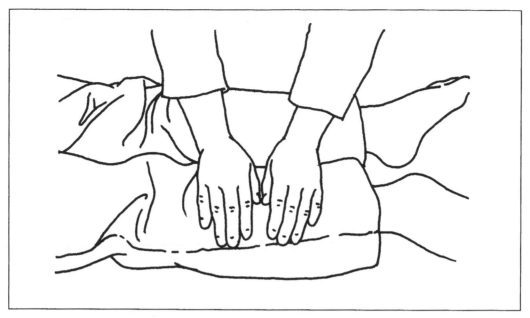

Position 15

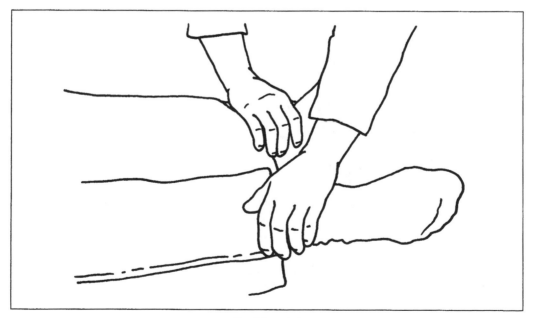

Position 16

Figure 4: Hand Positions for Treatment of Others (continued)

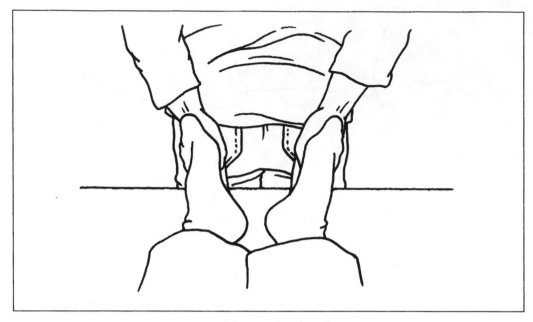

Position 17 (optional)

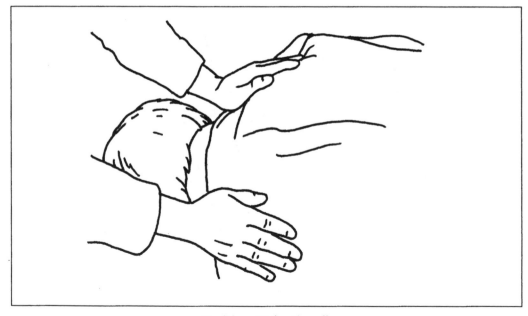

Position 18 (optional)

Figure 4: Hand Positions for Treatment of Others (continued)

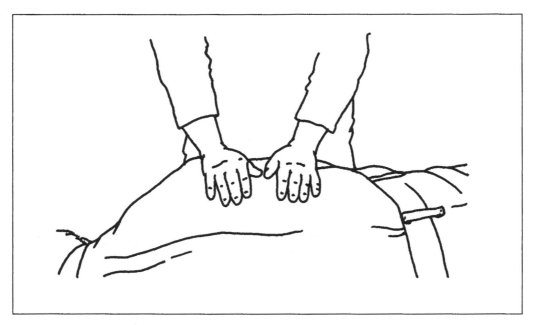

Position 19 (optional)

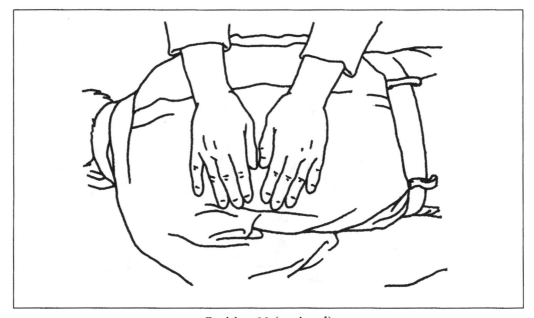

Position 20 (optional)

Figure 4: Hand Positions for Treatment of Others (continued)

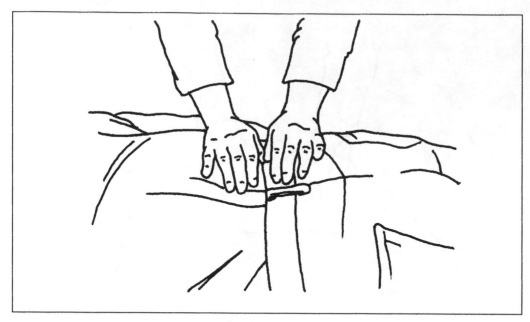

Position 21 (optional)

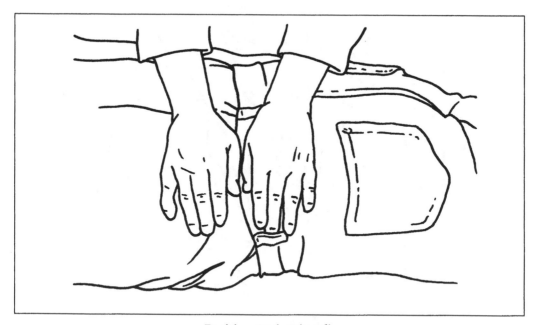

Position 22 (optional)

Figure 4: Hand Positions for Treatment of Others (continued)

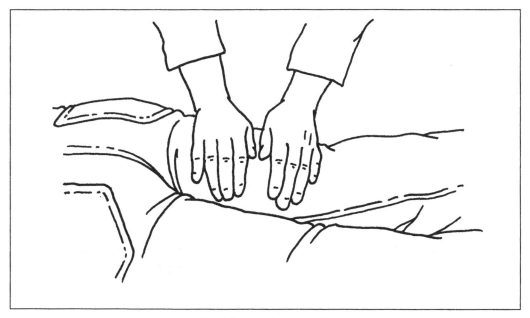

Position 23 (optional)

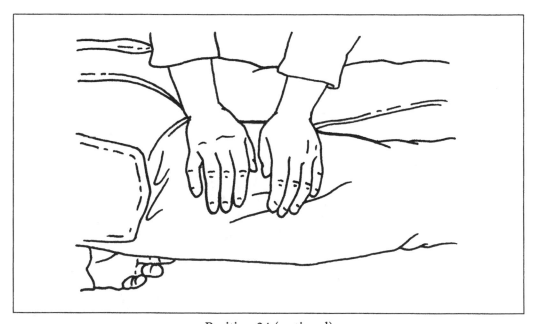

Position 24 (optional)

Figure 4: Hand Positions for Treatment of Others (continued)

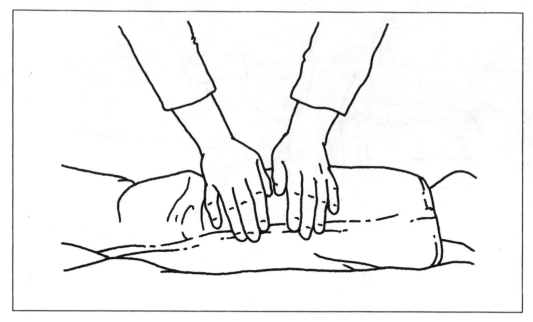

Position 25 (optional)

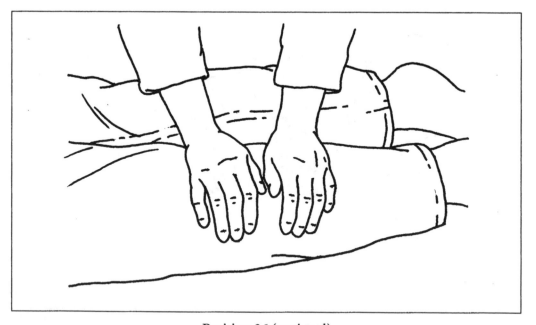

Position 26 (optional)

Figure 4: Hand Positions for Treatment of Others (continued)

Hand Positions

Reiki energy flows where it needs to go, in the physical body and in the subtle bodies. If I have an area in need of healing in my lower body, say my foot, and Reiki is done on my head, the energy will flow where it is needed for the highest good. It will flow through my body and go to my foot. Likewise, if I do Reiki for a bruise, but I really need to work on an emotional issue, it will flow to my emotional body rather than my physical body.

During the course of a healing session, it facilitates the process to place your hands directly on the area in need of healing. For specific ailments and injuries, you can start at the area of greatest concern. Simple and quick sessions can be done just on those areas. In most formal sessions, the practitioner will cover the body from head to toe, using various hand positions. Students speculate that Dr. Hayashi was the one who originated the hand positions, and recommended specific hand positions for specific ailments.

Modern Reiki practitioners usually start out learning the traditional hand positions, or a variation thereof, but then allow their intuition to guide them as they become more confident and comfortable doing healing sessions. Technically, you don't need to use the various hand positions or to move your hands at all, but they help provide a structure to the session when working on yourself or others.

According to traditional lore, the student should spend about five minutes on each position before moving on. I usually wait to feel the cycle of energy in my hands. Reiki energy can feel like heat, cold, tingles, prickliness, magnetism, or vibration. It builds in intensity and then winds down. It can last for thirty seconds or, in extreme cases, for more than ten minutes. As it winds down, I change positions, knowing the energy is done or the body is "full" in that position. If I don't move, the energy will build through another cycle, perhaps going to another part of the body, or the energy will simply shut off, so it does no harm in any case. If the Reiki flows, it is needed somewhere for the highest good. You don't control it, divine intelligence does. So go with it and follow your guidance.

To Touch or Not to Touch?

Although I initially learned Reiki as a form of hands-on healing, and explain it that way, a new movement has grown in the Reiki world called "hands-off" Reiki. Because of legal concerns regarding touch and body privacy issues, Reiki practitioners in certain areas practice Reiki without touch. They simply hold their hands over the body. I find it awkward personally, and I really feel touch is a component of the Reiki process. I may do Reiki with my hands off or slightly raised in sensitive areas, such as the throat or areas of body privacy, but most of the positions can be adapted to work around such issues. In the end, the choice is up to you as a practitioner, but I definitely prefer hands-on Reiki. People are often afraid to touch in our society, so I encourage this exchange of divine energy through the medium of physical contact.

When to Do Reiki

You can do Reiki whenever you want. Some feel restricted to the space of a formal healing session, but one of the benefits I find of Reiki versus traditional ritual magick is the easy access one has to the energy, without worry about imbalance or lack of concentration. The built-in safeguards of the Reiki attunement keep me from worrying about such problems.

Nothing has to be "wrong" for you to do Reiki. You don't have to have a major illness. It can be a simple "tune-up" to let the healing energy flow to maintain health. If the energy flows, then it is serving a higher good. If it doesn't, then you don't have to worry about it.

You can use it when you do have an imbalance, be it physical, mental, emotional, or spiritual. I do Reiki for aches and pains, illnesses, and in times of stress, conflict, or any emotional process that is revealing my issues and lessons to me. I try to do Reiki on myself everyday as a part of my spiritual practice.

Anytime you have a hand free, you can do Reiki, on yourself or on another who may need it. When I'm driving and resting one hand in my lap, I place the palm down on my thigh and let the Reiki flow. The same goes for watching television or movies and talking on the phone. When I'm with my partner, we can be hanging out on the couch or bed, but if I have a hand on him and the energy is needed, Reiki will flow. Usually we ask permission first, and I would inform any family member or friend that the Reiki is flowing, but we have so many personal exchanges already that I don't worry about compensation. Sometimes Reiki flow becomes such a normal part of life that you don't notice it much. My family members will point out to me when they feel the Reiki energy when we touch. I place my hands on my body when I meditate, making it a part of my spiritual practice. I even do Reiki in my sleep, going to bed or waking up with my hands on my body. Simply by placing my hands on my body, the Reiki flows. I can be conscious and fully aware, in meditation, or sleeping.

Reiki can be used on the go, in any situation where you think it will serve a good. You can offer it in the office, in the home, or wherever you are. When your hands are on, Reiki is on. There is no wrong way to do Reiki.

Reiki Sessions

Although Reiki can be done anywhere, anytime, for those in a professional context, a treatment session gives a format for the offering of Reiki. Such formats provide a comforting structure for both the practitioner and the recipient. Formats vary among traditions and practitioners. The following are some techniques that work well for me that I learned in the Reiki tradition.

Practical Points

Make sure you have taken care of all the practical considerations before the session begins. Make sure the room is set up. Have your massage table or chair set up. Make the space comfortable and clean. You can cleanse it through energy and scent with oils or incense. Change the sheets, blankets, or paper on your massage table. Clients also appreciate fresh breath. If you will need water, have it handy. Also have a glass of water ready for your client, either before or after the session.

Conversation

Take time to speak with your clients, explaining what Reiki is and isn't, and what to expect in a session with you. Ask them why they are here for a session, and what they hope to accomplish. Some Reiki practitioners use disclaimer or release forms. Now is the time to go over such legal agreements.

Intention

Help your client form a clear intention to set the tone of the session. Since we don't control Reiki, the result may be different from our intention, but setting an intention can help clients take responsibility for their own healing. (See the next paragraph for one method of setting an intention.)

Scanning

Scanning can help inspire an intention in a client. The hand chakras are very sensitive after an awakening in the attunement process, though many people can do this exercise without a Reiki attunement. Place your hands above the crown, and slowly move down over the chakras. Take notice of any differences in feeling, and where that feeling is. Differences may be in heat, temperature, energetic resistance, or density. Through intuition, determine what is the "normal" sensation for that person, at that time with you, and what differences indicate an abnormality or imbalance. Notice what body parts and chakras are associated with that area, and discuss the spiritual concepts associated with those parts when forming an intention with the client. Often what the client thinks he or she is there for, and what the Reiki is ready to work on, are two different things. Scanning can give us an idea of energetic health. In Japan, scanning is called Byosen.

Evocation

Although not a traditional part of a Reiki session, many practitioners use a spiritual evocation before doing a treatment, either silently or out loud, asking for spiritual guidance and aid for the session. You can state a general intent or specifically call upon beings such as spirit guides, angels, gods, or spiritual figures. I usually say out loud: "I offer this Reiki to you for the highest good, harming none, in balance with your intention. So mote it be." "So mote it be" means "It is so" in the Wiccan traditions. I can't resist adding elements of my Wiccan background to my sessions since many of my clients are witches, but you could just as easily say "So be it," "It is so," "Namaste," or even "Amen" at the end of that statement. Use whatever feels comfortable in your practice, or say it silently.

Grounding

Another Reiki "add-on" is the concept of grounding, found in most metaphysical traditions. Grounding is the act of putting yourself in your body, centered and stable. If you feel out of body, or off center, lightheaded, or overly energized, you might be ungrounded. Although Reiki's built-in safeguards protect you from the unwanted energies of your clients, some practitioners still feel off center or overwhelmed during a session. To ground yourself, imagine that your feet are like the roots of a tree, digging deep into the pure energy of the Earth, anchoring you here and now. Or imagine a beam of light, like an anchor, descending from the base of your spine down into the core of the Earth, tying you down as if you were a balloon weighted down.

Treatment

Make sure the client is as comfortable as possible on the treatment table. If lying down is not comfortable or possible for the recipient, Reiki can be given to a seated or standing client, though it can be more difficult and uncomfortable for the practitioner to give a full-body session. Once you are both prepared and the evocation has been offered in some way, begin your treatment using traditional or intuitive hand positions.

Sweeping and Smoothing

At the end of a session, modern practitioners will quickly move their hands from crown to feet over the recipient, approximately three times. They are sweeping away unwanted energies, as the energetic muck has been pushed to the surface. They are clearing it away. The motion imitates clearing off dirt and flinging it to the floor at the feet. The floor space is envisioned in a clearing white or violet light, or a prayer is said to ask the world to transmute the energy. I know a practitioner who has a bowl of sea salt and water at the end of the table. Salt is known for its cleansing properties. Harmful energy is automatically drawn to it and absorbed by its crystalline structure. The practitioner then replaces the water after each session. The final motion is to smooth down the aura and return it to a normal level of openness. Since the chakras "open" and the aura expands during a session, the smoothing process brings them back to a normal waking level, helping ground the recipient.

Final Blessing and Conversation

Treatments end with a blessing or thank you, silently or out loud, much like the evocation. Taking a cue from my teachers, I usually say: "We are both blessed by the gifts of Reiki. Namaste." Sometimes I sneak in a Wiccan "Blessed be" if I know the client is comfortable with it. I then like to spend some time speaking with the recipient, sharing my impressions and most importantly, hearing about his or her impressions.

Exercise: Self-Scanning

Try doing a scan on yourself. It can be difficult, because we have expectations about our health and often cannot see improvements or problems if we don't expect them. But if you approach it with an open mind, you can receive great information before things become a problem.

Get into a meditative state, and try either of these techniques. The first possibility is to quietly and slowly run your hands from the crown to the groin, seeking to feel different sensations, as you would with a client. The other possibility, if you are visually oriented, is to hold the intention of seeing yourself and your chakras in your mind's eye, as if you were holding a mirror, and then take notice of what seems to be balanced and what is out of balance.

When done, you can focus your Reiki self-treatments on the areas of your body where you are out of balance.

Sense of Style

Everybody has a different sense of style, including Reiki practitioners. Although the different traditions set up a format and a set of procedures as guidelines, each Reiki practitioner has their own sense of execution. Some are more mystically oriented, and set the tone of the room with ceremonial items, incense, and candles. As someone who is more magickally oriented and comfortable using ritual and guided imagery, I often guide my clients through a relaxation and meditation to help open them to their own inner spiritual guidance. Other practitioners are more clinical. Some like to talk before and after, while others strictly do Reiki, with little discussion.

Many people come to Reiki class with some intuitive or psychic abilities. Students often report an increase or opening of these abilities after an attunement, but that is not a specific intention of the initiation, just an occasional side benefit. It can be hard to deal with psychic information during a session. Some practitioners focus on it and make it a part of their style, while others ignore it. I tend to use psychic impressions during the scanning process and then share my impressions and feelings after the session. I have practitioner friends who are very psychic, who ask questions of the client during the session to get to core issues. I prefer to give clients an inner experience first and ask questions later. Style and technique will vary among practitioners. I've learned as much while getting Reiki sessions from others as I have from taking classes and doing treatments. Explore the many styles of Reiki.

You Are a Healing Facilitator, Not a God!

One of the most important things to remember when doing Reiki is that you are a healing facilitator. It's easy to get hooked into the title and role of a "healer." I use that word because people identify with it, but in essence I mean a "healing facilitator." No one heals anyone else. Healers simply provide an opportunity to heal and help one through the process. Even modern medical practitioners, doctors, and nurses help others heal. They provide the body with the necessary structure, nutrition, or chemicals to heal, but the body ends up healing itself. As Reiki practitioners, we provide the necessary energy and help others come into an awareness, but they must heal themselves. We cannot fix them or do it for them, even though that is the model we have in the medical community. In the end, no one can fix us. We must take care of the roots of our imbalances, or they will come back to haunt us. Just because you have access to the Reiki system doesn't mean that you necessarily have all the answers for your clients or an absolute cure for what is ailing them. Like many in the medical profession, it is easy to get a sense of power from our work and think we are somehow better than others because of it. Ultimately, Reiki is not about power, it's about service.

Healing Crisis

Earlier in this chapter, we talked about both the practitioner's cleansing process after the attunement and the recipient's cleansing. When I first describe the cleansing process to prospective clients, I describe it as a "healing awareness." But when you are on the receiving end of this awareness, it is more aptly named a "healing crisis" by practitioners. A thorough Reiki teacher will explore the concepts of release, awareness, and crisis with students. I didn't have such a background when I experienced my first healing crisis.

I first got involved in Reiki to help my mother with a pain in her leg. Magick, witchcraft, and crystals were not working, and a good friend told us about Reiki. My mother didn't want to travel to the class, so I said I would take it and then be able to "do Reiki" for her.

At first, the results were phenomenal. Her pain was relieved completely for hours. But when the treatment "wore off," she was in worse pain then when we started. The only advice I got from others was to continue to do Reiki, and it was the right advice. Her body and energy, subconsciously, were holding on to the energy block. We all hold on to things that are familiar to us. Though we may consciously want to heal and change, it can be a fearsome prospect, so parts of us resist unknowingly. The energy will flush out the "mud" when it's ready to go. All you can do is make the energy available, and help the recipient examine the thoughts and feelings that may be holding back the process.

Not being versed in the thoughts and feelings that can arise during a healing session, but only the physical aspects of Reiki, I thought I was causing my mother's pain. At the time, practitioners in the medical community were not as familiar with Reiki as they are now. When we went for medical help, the nurse practitioner said something like, "Hmm . . . Reiki. We don't know much about that. It could be causing more harm than good. We just don't know enough about it or how it works." She scared me, and we stopped doing Reiki, and the block remained for quite a while.

In retrospect, I should have continued doing Reiki and allowed the process to resolve itself. But we both let fear rule us. If I had been familiar with the concept of the healing crisis on the physical, emotional, mental, and spiritual levels, it might have been different. Now, being aware of it, and making my clients aware of it, we can take the healing to deeper levels and work with our energy on all levels of awareness.

Reiki Lineage

The last aspect of the First Degree is sharing Reiki lineage. In some ways, Reiki is like a family, and we all trace ourselves back to the same spiritual forefather, Dr. Usui. All Reiki practitioners in this system can trace their connection back to Dr. Usui. Like many magickal orders and covens, practitioners often feel it is important to know where the energy of the lineage originated, and who brought it into being. Others don't really care where the Reiki came from, because Reiki is simply Reiki, regardless of the source. I like to know where things originated for my own personal study, and to be able to share this information with my students, but in the end, I agree: Reiki is simply Reiki and that is the most important thing to me.

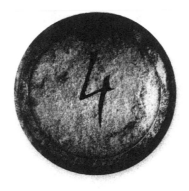

The Second Degree: Reiki Two

While the first level of Reiki instruction focuses on the earthy foundations and the hands-on practice of Reiki, the second level stresses a more mental and emotional component. At this level, not only are concepts beyond the traditional in-person approach discussed, but techniques based upon these more esoteric concepts are put into practice. With an emphasis on the concept of sacred symbols conveying the power of Reiki and the possibility of healing beyond space and even time, teachers often lose the conventional, nonmystical student. But for those interested in exploring such realms, Reiki Two opens up a whole new world.

In my Reiki Two experience, I really awakened to the energy as part of my spiritual path, and not just as a simple tool or technique to try when my other magickal healing abilities had failed or were not applicable. I saw that the concepts behind Reiki were similar to my own experiences in the traditions of magick, and could appreciate Reiki more because of my previous magickal training. Also, Reiki Two helped dismiss my sense that there is an unknowable mystery to Reiki that is only reserved for Reiki Masters, and left me feeling that I was really part of the tradition. I think this was in large part due to the open and welcoming nature of my fairly nontraditional teacher as much as the material presented in Reiki Two.

The Sacred Symbols

An important part of the level two instruction is the concept of Reiki symbols. The Reiki symbols are like keys that are used to convey the energy of Reiki to clients during healing sessions, and also to attune and transfer the energy from teacher to student in the teaching process.

Think of each symbol as a key, or portal, to an aspect of the universal life force. When you activate the symbol, you are calling upon that aspect of the energy. Each symbol has its own individual character or flavor, its own use and purpose in the art of Reiki.

A practitioner can activate the symbols in a variety of ways, including drawing, visualizing, intending, or chanting. The various traditions teach specific ways to activate the symbols using a combination of these techniques, but in the end, intention is the most important component.

Through the use of the three practitioner symbols taught in Reiki Two, one can achieve a variety of effects, such as energy boosts, emotional and mental balance, distance healing, and healing the past. These symbols opened the link to magick for me. Both magick and Reiki use symbols to activate specific intentions. In the most modern traditions, the symbols are used ritualistically for a variety of purposes that are not specifically healing, such as cleansing the energy of a room or manifesting a personal intention.

Does "Sacred" Equal "Secret"?

Here we come upon one of the most controversial parts of Reiki history, one to which I gave much serious thought before writing this book. In the most traditional lineages, the symbols are considered quite a serious matter and not to be discussed with any outsiders to the Reiki lineage, even those initiates below the second level. The traditional names are not to be spoken, only the purpose names, such as Power symbol or Distance symbol. They are not to be shown to others.

Extreme traditions don't allow the symbols to be written down, and when they are drawn in order to be learned in class practice, the papers are collected and ritually burned once memorized. Because of this practice, the symbols have changed in form over the years, and without a definitive standard available, many variations of the symbols exist. After Hawayo Takata's death, her Reiki Master students discovered that they had different versions of the same symbols. Each version worked, proving that the intention and meaning behind the symbols is more important than the symbols themselves. Less extreme traditions allow you to have copies of the symbols, but they are not to be shown or redrawn in ink. They are only to be drawn in the air, on the roof of your mouth with your tongue, or with your eyes. The most modern traditions don't care how you use the symbols, as long as you remember them and use them in your healing work.

The heart of the disagreement over symbol use is the age-old question "Does *sacred* mean *secret*?" The symbols were kept hidden out of respect for their sacredness. But the effort required to keep them hidden, and the apparent price tag that went along with them, made people in some Reiki traditions question the practice of absolute secrecy. It appeared that the absolute secrecy of the estoric symbols increased their financial value, and some were charging large fees for the training that revealed these symbols. Just because something is revealed to others doesn't make it less sacred. Something can be known and still be treated with respect. If Reiki is universal, shouldn't we all have access to it?

If you are not attuned to Reiki energy by a Reiki Master, the symbols will not work for you. If you see the symbols, you may think that you have the Reiki system attunement, but you will not have the safeguards that come with it. Some people will then attempt to do a healing, by using the symbols directly or believing that because they have seen the symbols, they are attuned. Since they are not attuned to Reiki, or do not have knowledge of other safe and effective traditions of hands-on healing, they end up using their own personal energy in the healing and are left weakened and suseptible to illness. I agree that this scenario is a potential danger, but I don't see any inherent harm in letting others see the symbols. In fact, they will either have a helpful effect or no effect at all. A few practitioners I know give the symbols to clients to meditate on between sessions. Dr. Usui wasn't attuned by a Reiki Master. He studied the symbols and had a personal, meditative exchange with the energy that the symbols embodied during his retreat. I don't expect that too many people will have Dr. Usui's experience, but I don't pretend to be the final judge on that.

Another concern is that the Reiki symbols could be misused or used for harm, as some people claim they have in the past in the ancient world, like in some versions of the story of Atlantis. They were kept secret because they are so powerful. Well, if you listened to the first argument, then you know that the symbols would have no effect if the person had not been attuned to them by a Reiki Master. If the person had been attuned, then all the safeguards would be in place for the person to be guided by higher will, making misuse impossible. If they are symbols from a system of healing guided by higher will, then how can they be used for harm? In my opinion, they can't. Energy can be used for harm, but not as accessed through the Reiki symbols. This concern grows out of people's fear of losing control of something they never really controlled in the first place.

Now that the symbols have been revealed in other books and websites, they are still sacred and they still work. Reiki Masters haven't noticed a diminishment of the Reiki energy. In fact, the opposite has happened: the flow seems to be getting stronger as more people tune into it to heal the world.

As you might have guessed, I fall in the camp that believes that sacred doesn't necessarily mean secret, and vice versa. There are many sacred texts that are available to the general public, and it does not diminish their sacredness one iota. For example, the Bible is sacred to many, and is readily available in many languages.

We live in an age where secrets are being revealed to all. Sacred information that was previously kept hidden, particularly in the West, is now more accessible. In our culture, we have an influx of esoteric lore being made public. Look in any bookstore and you will find the once-hidden knowledge of meditation, healing, yoga, martial arts, astrology, and other esoteric sciences and arts.

Reiki Two Practitioner Symbols

For each of the three Reiki practitioner symbols, a traditional way to draw them is given in this section. Variations on the "correct" way to draw them are as numerous as the symbol variations themselves. Although I teach them the way I learned them, if you find a way that is better for you, then use it.

I draw symbols with both my first and second fingers. I learned it this way to keep a balanced polarity, and I like it, but I know many who draw them with only one finger. I usually draw the symbols with my fingers first, using the traditional drawing instructions. I then activate the symbol by chanting its name three times, silently or out loud, while I push the symbol into the body with my fingers three times as I chant. You can also draw the symbols with your whole fist, your eye movement, or your tongue on the roof of your mouth, or you can simply visualize them whole. If you use a variation of the traditional drawings shown here, I think it will still be effective, though some teachers believe that drawing them in the correct pattern is the only effective technique. I teach them the way I learned them, but there are many variations. No one can say that one way is absolutely right. You can chant the symbol names with intention, and not

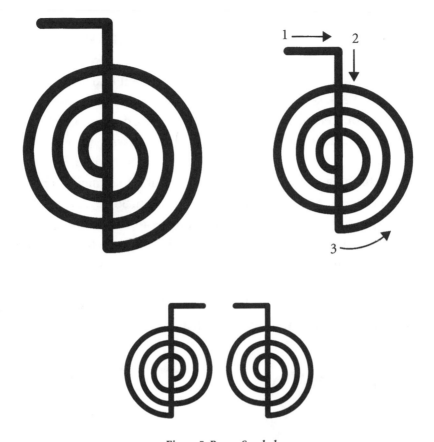

Figure 5: Power Symbol

specifically draw them in the air, though practitioners in the more conservative Reiki traditions would find this idea unacceptable.

Now, without further ado, I share with you the magickal energy of the three Reiki Two practitioner symbols.

Power Symbol

Cho Ku Rei (pronounced "cho-koo-ray") literally means "Put the power here" or "Increase the power." I think of it as an "on" switch for Reiki. Traditional Japanese Reiki Masters translate this symbol to mean "Focus." Practitioners often say its name silently before all uses of Reiki, or draw it on their hands before all sessions. I do this sometimes, but not always.

Cho Ku Rei increases the power and flow of Reiki whenever used. It can be drawn with the spiral counterclockwise, its original form, or clockwise. Magickal practitioners often feel the clockwise version is more powerful, or adds power, while the counterclockwise version removes unwanted energy; but if the intent is to increase power, either version will work. The clockwise movement, called deosil in Wicca, is used to increase or build energy. The counterclockwise movement, called widdershins in Wicca, is used to decrease energy or banish. In magickal training, the clockwise movement follows the motion of the Sun as it casts a shadow. Following the Sun's movement is symbolic of health and growth. To move against the Sun's movement is to diminish. Though this is a useful magickal concept, it is not an inherent part of Reiki. Some magickal Reiki practitioners use the two different versions of Cho Ku Rei with the clockwise/counterclockwise intentions in mind. Use your intuition as to which version to use. Neither can do any harm. Use this symbol anytime you would like during a session, on a particular body part or drawn down the body. I draw the vertical line down the chakra column, with the flag at the crown and the end of the vertical line at the root. Then I draw the spiral around the body. I often start and end a session with Cho Ku Rei.

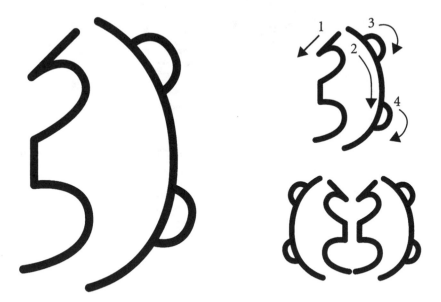

Figure 6: Mental/Emotional Symbol

Mental/Emotional Symbol

Sei He Ki (pronounced "say-hay-key") activates your divine presence. Use this symbol to balance your mind and emotions, male and female energies, and left and right brains, especially when drawn doubled over the head or the entire body, in a mirror image (see figure 6). The single version is also very powerful for balance. Sei He Ki heals anger, depression, sadness, fear, and addictions—any difficult feelings or thoughts. Almost all disease has a mental/emotional root, so it is a powerful symbol for getting to the root of a problem. Use Sei He Ki to activate the unconscious mind, to empower daily affirmations, and to find lost objects. This symbol, like Cho Ku Rei, clears unwanted energy. When doing a full-body treatment, I discuss a good affirmation with the client before starting. During the treatment, I imagine a door with Sei He Ki on it that leads to the subconscious. I then open the door, and place any affirmations into the mind by chanting "Sei He Ki, (Affirmation), Sei He Ki" three times. Traditional Japanese Reiki practitioners call it the Harmony symbol.

Distance Symbol

Hon Sha Ze Sho Nen (pronounced "hone-sha-zay-show-nen") heals beyond space and time, working on all levels and dimensions. All time is one time, and Reiki healings go beyond our linear time. This symbol is the focus for distant treatments, creating a bridge across space and time to safely send the energy, but it can also be used for in-person treatments to great effect. Draw Hon Sha Ze Sho Nen from head to toe to send the healing across space and time, so it is not limited to the time of your individual session. The healing will move toward completion, beyond the boundary of the physical session. Many claim that it helps heal the karma of the client. I don't think of karma as something that needs to be healed, but the symbol can bring awareness and understanding of the past to bring healing in the present and future.

Distance Treatments

Apart from the symbols of the Second Degree, the main goal of this level is to learn the art of distance Reiki treatments. The concept behind distance healing is that the universal life force is a field of energy, connecting all things. There is no distance in the universal life field. We are all one. To the Eastern mystic, separation is the illusion, the Maya.

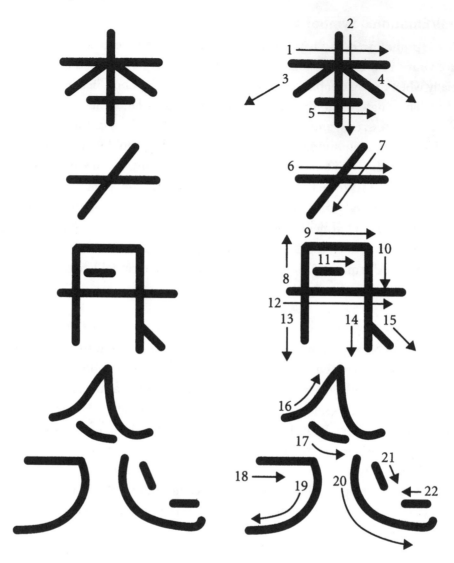

Figure 7: Distance Symbol

The truth is, we are all one, we are all connected, and enlightenment is the process of seeing through the illusion and living from the truth. To the Western magician or witch, the same concept is held in the Hermetic Principle of Mentalism. We are all thoughts in the divine mind. We are all smaller parts of the larger whole, never separate. Our own thoughts appear to be individual to us, but they are a part of the greater mental body. We also appear to be individual, but we are part of the larger divine being—God, Goddess, Great Spirit—whatever you choose to call it. Scientists call this the holographic model of the universe.

In theory, this field of universal life force not only breaks all distance barriers, but also all time barriers, and the distance healing technique can be used to heal across time, into the past. The symbol used in the technique, Hon Sha Ze Sho Nen, is usually translated as "No past, no present, no future," which means "No time, no space. All is one."

The distance healing technique in Reiki is remarkably easy to learn. What I really love about this technique, versus other techniques of magickal or psychic healing that I've learned, is its simplicity. You don't have to be skilled in visualization, sensing energy, or spell work to use it. Many people mistakenly think that only "special," "magickal," or "psychic" practitioners can do such healing work. But in Reiki Two, students learn that anyone in tune with the Reiki energy can do distance healing with the symbol and technique. Through the energetic link created by the Distance symbol, they often get intuitive or psychic impressions even though they don't consider themselves psychic. Through trust in the Reiki energy and the technique, their confidence and abilities expand. Through Reiki, we can all discover that we are special, magickal, and psychic.

Like all things magickal, and all things in Reiki, there are variations in the technique among individual traditions and teachers. Later in this section, I present the versions that I teach and use in my own practice.

Certain traditions say that this distance healing technique doesn't work unless you have had your second attunement, but I feel that it still works with only the first attunement. You have this Distance symbol in your energy field after the first attunement, so in theory it should work after any Reiki attunement.

Before you do a distance healing session, ask permission of the recipient if possible. You can explain what a distance Reiki session is to the recipient however you like. Some describe it as plainly as possible, while others describe it as a kind of healing "prayer." If you can't get conscious permission and still feel called to do a distance Reiki session, you can ask permission of the recipient's higher self as you start the distance healing session.

Sit down comfortably and take a few deep breaths to center yourself. You don't have to be in a meditative state or completely peaceful to do it. The Reiki energy flows through you. You are not using your energy to heal. But a little focus helps you remember the technique.

Think about the person to whom you want to send Reiki energy. You don't have to visualize the recipient, though that doesn't hurt. Some of the techniques stress visualization, which makes it impossible for the practitioner to send Reiki to someone without a clear idea of how the person looks, but I've found that unnecessary. The intention is the most important thing. You don't have to say the recipient's name, though that can help make a connection. Simply think of the person. Hold the intention that you would like to send this person Reiki.

Draw the Distance symbol in the air in front of you, as if you were drawing on a blackboard. Draw the symbol and then activate it by saying its name (Hon Sha Ze Sho Nen) out loud or silently, three times. This creates a gateway between you and the recipient, across space and time. Think of the recipient. That's all it takes to make the connection.

If you don't have the conscious permission of the recipient, ask the recipient's higher self. The higher self refers to the spiritual, divine self. Ceremonial magick traditions see it as the angelic self, calling it the Holy Guardian Angel. This is the part of a person that is in tune with the divine mind and the individual's path. If the person is ill or injured, and the illness or injury is serving the person for a higher good, then the Reiki will not affect the illness and you will either get a "No" response or the energy will go toward the person's emotional, mental, or spiritual healing.

Say to yourself: "I ask the higher self of (Recipient's name) for permission to do this Reiki healing." Simply go by your gut instincts as to whether you feel a yes or a no response. Certain Reiki practitioners use a pendulum or muscle testing to get a response, but I go by my intuition. If I am unsure about the answer, or feel that I might be letting my ego (what I want) rather than the higher good answer, I hold this intention: "I ask for this Reiki to be used for the highest good, and if it is not for the highest good of (Recipient's name), I ask it go wherever it is needed, or to the Earth herself."

Here are several different ways to perform a distance healing session. Practitioners should be versed in all of them, but will usually favor one or two in their personal practice.

Surrogate

I imagine the energy or image of the recipient, the size of a doll, coming through the "blackboard" where I drew the Distance symbol. Then I place that energy into a surrogate, such as a pillow or teddy bear. Then I do Reiki on this miniature client. I handle it just like a regular session, scanning and using the symbols. I may not do all the hand positions, since my hands are larger on this surrogate, but during the distance session, the flow of energy from my hands may last longer in a single position than it would during an in-person treatment. I do Reiki on the entire body with just a few positions. When I am done, I sweep away the unwanted released energy and neutralize it. Then I imagine lifting the energy out of the surrogate and sending it through the blackboard and back to the client. I then wipe the Distance symbol off the imaginary board and say a final blessing, as I would at the end of a regular session.

Self Surrogate

The self surrogate is the same as the previous technique, but instead of placing the energy of the client into a pillow or stuffed animal, it is put into the practitioner's body. You can put a miniature image of the client into your leg, intending the person's head at your knee and the feet at your hips. You can also imagine the recipient in your entire body. As you do a "self" treatment, you are actually sending Reiki to the recipient over a distance, using your own body like a giant doll. People get nervous about this technique because so many healing traditions warn the practitioner about taking on the illness or emotions of the client. I agree, but Reiki energy flows one-way. You cannot take on the illnesses of others through this technique, using the Distance symbol. You are simply using your body as a place to put your hands to send the energy.

Visualization

Visualization techniques can be done in several ways. I often use visualization in conjunction with the surrogate technique. If I don't have a pillow or other suitable vessel available, I visualize a doll-sized image of the recipient between my hands, floating in the air. I prefer visualization to the self surrogate technique, but that's just me. Both work. I used this visualization technique with a friend of mine who was passing on in the hospital. His family members wanted to be close to him, so even though I wasn't able to touch him, I was still able to do Reiki. You can also visualize yourself going to the recipient and doing a full-body session in your mind. Or you can visualize bringing the recipient to you, to your own Reiki table or into a Reiki room in your mind's eye, where you do the session. Both work, though some practitioners feel they can't do this technique if they can't visualize the intended "target."

Symbols

Once you open the gateway between yourself and the recipient, you can simply draw and activate various combinations of Reiki symbols, as intuitively guided, on the surrogate, just as you would if you were there in person. You do this without actually laying your hands on anything or even visualizing hands-on techniques. You simply use the symbols.

Beaming

Beaming is the process of sending Reiki at a distance, but through a line of sight, visualizing a beam of Reiki as light emanating from the hands, heart, or eyes to the recipient. This technique doesn't require creating a gateway through the Distance symbol.

Intention/Prayer

When you can't do a full distance session, you can simply intend through prayer and focused will to send Reiki energy to the recipient, without any fancy techniques, symbols, or hand positions. Though this technique works, I use it the least because I like to connect with and have an experience with the recipient, and be able to share my impressions.

When doing a distance healing, practitioners often set up an "appointment" when the recipient will be in a quiet space, inviting the healing to occur. Though it can be great to engage the recipient to be aware and hold their own intentions of healing, it is not necessary. Practitioners talk about how it can be dangerous to send Reiki if they don't know what the recipient is doing. They fear that if the person is driving, the Reiki could make them relax so much that they get into an accident. I've never had that happen. Reiki cannot be used for harm, so if the recipient's higher self feels it would be harmful, the reception of it will be delayed until a more appropriate time. Reiki moves across time as well as space.

You can do distance Reiki on animals, plants, towns, cities, countries, disaster zones, and even the entire planet. No past, no present, no future, no limits!

Detachment

Detachment is one of the greatest gifts I have received in Reiki, and I stress its importance in the Second Degree. Through Reiki, we are not attached to the result or outcome. We may have an intention, but we don't need to feel responsible for the outcome. We offer our time to be a vessel for the energy. We become a flute to be played by the divine, the unseen hand. When you apply certain aspects of detachment to everyday life, you can see how great a blessing Reiki can be in all areas, even beyond healing.

When a practitioner is really attached to the result of a Reiki session, the energy doesn't seem to flow as easily. Sometimes the less a practitioner pays attention, the stronger the energy flows. I was aghast to hear my teacher tell me that some of her best sessions occurred while she was mentally creating her grocery list or reflecting on her "to do" list. I thought that a practitioner should be fully present and worry about the client. But she wasn't worried. She let Reiki do its thing. She was as present as she needed to be, but unattached to what she thought the result should be. She didn't hold a final outcome in her mind, and simply let the Reiki flow. Now, in my own practice, I must say that I agree with her. Some of my best sessions for the client have been when I've been the most detached.

To help with detachment in the personal healing process, I suggest to students to do a distance Reiki treatment on themselves. The process of doing Reiki on yourself over a "distance" can help you gain a new perspective, and see your issues and problems in a more detached and less personal way. It can also help you develop greater unconditional love and compassion for yourself, without the personal attachment.

Growing as a Healing Facilitator

I always end my Reiki Two course with a discussion about becoming a healing facilitator, focusing on the mental and emotional components of being a practitioner. We talk in-depth about emotional release, ranging from intense crying to deep laughter while a client is on the table. We also talk about using breath work to relax a client. By overemphasizing your breath, a client will usually subconsciously match your breath. If you notice someone getting tense or preparing for a release, you can help them breathe through it by deep breathing. We also discuss grounding techniques, such as energy work, guided visualization, and grounding stones like smoky quartz and hematite, to bring a client back to the present.

Other healing modalities, combined with Reiki, such as massage, crystal healing, flower essences, aromatherapy, toning, meditation, and hypnotherapy, are discussed as complementary techniques. I also work with spirit guides and aura gazing in my own work, and delve into them with my students. Such techniques and tools will be explored in later chapters as part of the expanded magickal view of Reiki. As a class, we work though interview and discussion techniques for dealing with clients. Throughout the process, the intention is to guide the Reiki student away from thinking solely about the body and healing the physical, and to bring more awareness to the mental and emotional aspects of healing with others. In Reiki, we learn to honor the whole person, not just the body.

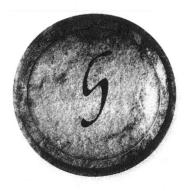

The Third Degree: Reiki Master

While Reiki One has a physical emphasis and Reiki Two has a mental and emotional component, Reiki Three focuses on the spiritual path of Reiki. Usually termed the Master level, here the initiate learns a greater awareness of Reiki, the spiritual path and principles involved in it, and the path of service to others, as a more experienced practitioner and as a teacher, helping empower other practitioners.

What Is a Reiki Master?

What is a Reiki Master? Ask a Reiki Master that question, and you will probably get as many different answers as you have Reiki Masters. The experience and practice of the third level varies among traditions and teachers. It is a very individual process. But in the course of the conversation, you will find two distinct schools of thought regarding the title Reiki Master.

In the original traditions of Usui Reiki, the practice is divided into three levels: two practitioner levels and the final Master level. The word master literally means "teacher," as translated from the Japanese. When you say Reiki Master, more accurately you mean

Reiki teacher. A Reiki Master must not only know the material and embody it in life to present to others, but must also have the knowledge and ability to pass energetic attunements to the student, so the student can be initiated into Reiki.

The last level of Reiki training requires a big financial investment as well as a level of dedication that almost requires new Reiki Masters to dedicate their entire lives to Reiki. Since each attunement comes with a spiritual awakening or cleanse, as well as an increased ability to channel energy, students wanted to receive the energy of the third level, but had no desire to teach or pass attunements. Western Reiki Masters divided the Master level into two sublevels to accommodate this desire.

The first sublevel includes a Master attunement and training in what are called "advanced" practitioner techniques, in anything from shamanism and psychic surgery to crystal healing. This first sublevel is called Reiki IIIa or Advanced Reiki Training, among other titles. Reiki IIIb became the teacher training, and usually includes another Master attunement, training in the process of passing attunements, teaching curriculum, business practices, and often an apprenticeship program.

As human nature will have it, people often want a title to accompany the level of accomplishment they have reached. Some graduates of the first sublevel were called Reiki III Practitioners, but somehow, eventually, the title Reiki Master was used, and the Reiki IIIb graduates were distinguished as Reiki Master/Teachers. In reality, that's like saying Reiki Teacher/Teacher. Unfortunately, many at the IIIa level misunderstood what a Reiki Master was, as the teaching of Usui changed and mutated with New Age mysticism. I don't think there's anything wrong with such mating. I've benefited from it greatly, but I think a good teacher, and tradition, makes it clear what is traditional Reiki and what is an "add on" to the traditional practice.

A small number of these new Reiki "Masters" sometimes confuse the title that was meant to mean "teacher" with "spiritual master" or "ascended master," meaning a person who has transcended the polarities or karma of normal human consciousness and has moved to another, more enlightened level of consciousness. I've heard people say that their Reiki Three attunement "grounded" their karma and they were awakened as enlightened masters. The third attunement is very spiritual and can awaken the receiver to a whole new world, but it is not an instant, easy-open package to enlightenment. If anything, the Reiki Three cleanse can bring up a lot of issues that need to be healed. It can be a very difficult, taxing process that lasts for many months or years, and it doesn't result in automatic enlightenment. If you are to relate the word Master to spiritual master, the title should remind the Reiki teacher to continually aspire to be a spiritual master, but it does not confer instant spiritual mastery.

Even when not taken to such an extreme, the concept of a Reiki Master as a teacher is sometimes greatly misunderstood. I had an experience where someone asked me what my Reiki training was. When I replied "Reiki Master," her response was, "Oh. So you don't teach it. You're just a Reiki Master." Another person told a newly graduated Reiki Master of my tradition that she was robbed by me, because everyone knows there are really four levels of Reiki, not just three. Since the third level has been broken into two levels by so many traditions without clear distinctions, we as a community may need to have to rethink our choice of words and titles.

I'm not big on titles in general, and often just drop the word Master in favor of Reiki teacher. The word teacher doesn't come with as much baggage as the word Master, and I'm not really attached to an identity as a Reiki Master. In the Shamballa Reiki tradition, level three is called Master-Healer or Master-Practitioner. The next level is distinct, called level four, and is given the title Master-Teacher. The word Master is reserved for those who want to use it, but it makes a clear distinction between a practitioner and a teacher. In the end, titles, certificates, and lineages don't matter as much as the work people do with the energy itself.

The Mysterious Master Symbols

The Master symbols are set apart from the first three practitioner symbols because they are essential in the attunement process. Some Reiki Masters only use them in the attunement process. I find them powerful both in attunements, in sessions, and in my personal life. The purpose of the Master symbols is to open the physical and spiritual bodies to the energy of Reiki, and to open the recipient's consciousness to divine will, the divine higher guidance that directs the Reiki energy.

Traditional Master Symbol

The traditional Master symbol in the Usui system of Reiki is called Di Ko Myo, pronounced "die-koe-me-oh." Consisting of a stylized Japanese kanji script, Di Ko Myo is usually translated as "Treasure house of great beaming light, great bright Sun and Moon, shine on me" or "Great Being of the Universe, shine on me, be my friend." I've always found that second translation funny, since in some schools of metaphysical healing, you make contact with a healing spirit guide or angel, and that spirit acts as the source of your healing energy, instead of your personal energy. Could Reiki be the same concept, but with a more universal being? Perhaps so.

There are several variations of this symbol. It is used primarily in attunements to connect the recipient to the Reiki energy and the higher self. It can also be used in healing sessions, drawn in a specific place in need of healing, or down the entire body, to facilitate the Reiki healing process. To differentiate it from the next symbol, I learned to chant this Master symbol as "Usui Di Ko Myo" to activate it.

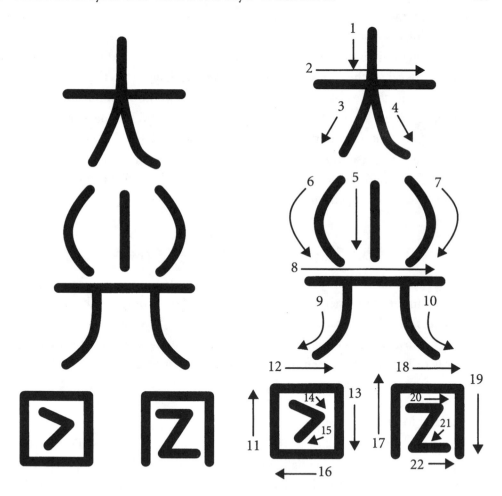

Figure 8: Traditional Master Symbol

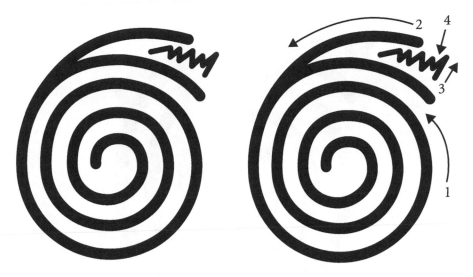

Figure 9: Tibetan Master Symbol

Tibetan Master Symbol

Di Ko Myo, or Di Ko Mio, is considered the Tibetan Master symbol, though there are conflicting reports as to how it came into the modern Reiki traditions. In the Shamballa Reiki tradition, it is called the Atlantean Master symbol. It is also referred to as Dumo. Two primary versions of it exist, and I use the first personally (figures 9 and 10). The form of this symbol seems much more similar to the primal nature of the Power symbol and the Mental-Emotional symbol than the Japanese styling of the Distance and Traditional Master symbols. In many ways, it seems like a combination of the Power symbol and the Grounding symbol, which is presented later in this chapter. In the Tibetan traditions of Reiki, this symbol is used as part of the Violet Breath/Dragon Breath attunement process, described later in this chapter. Like the traditional version of the Master symbol, it can be used in both attunements and healing sessions. I use it on all the chakras, to align them with the highest consciousness and to me. It seems to act as a spiritual "rotor-rooter," clearing all energy points and dissolving all blocks. When you meditate on the symbol, it appears to be a funneling vortex of energy with a bolt of lightning connecting the heavens and earth. Many teachers completely substitute the Tibetan symbol for the Traditional symbol, because it is easier to remember and draw.

Practitioners of certain Reiki traditions state that this symbol should not be used in healing. It will work, but the healer then assumes responsibility for the recipient's healing. This makes no sense. When you consider the metaphysical principles involved in Reiki, such statements cannot be true.

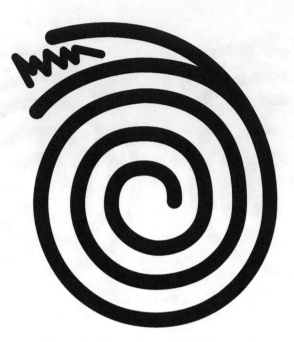

Figure 10: Tibetan Master Symbol Reversed

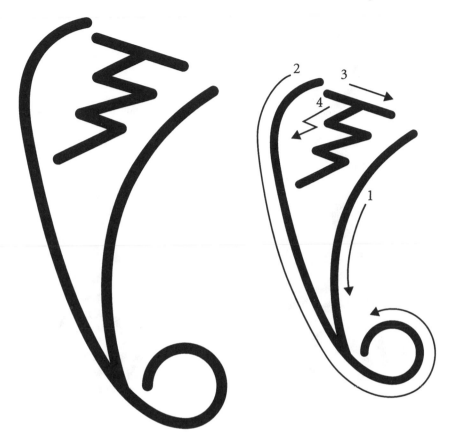

Figure 11: Alternate Tibetan Master Symbol

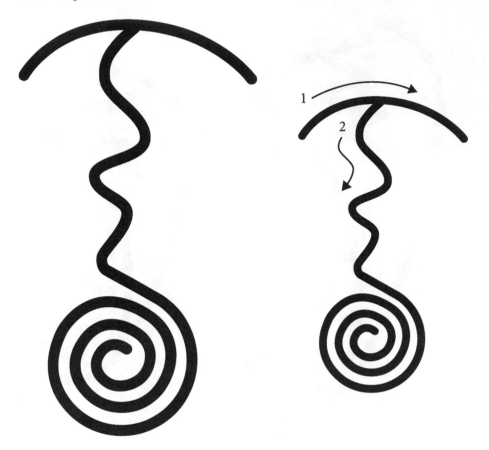

Figure 12: Serpent of Fire

Serpent of Fire

Nin Giz Zida (pronounced "nin-geez-zee-da") is another symbol attributed to Tibet. Called the Serpent of Fire, it is used to align the chakras and energy system to prepare a student for the attunement, or to prepare a client for the healing session. The serpent imagery is reminiscent of the kundalini, the fiery serpent energy of the Hindu traditions. This energy is said to be coiled in the root chakra to be awakened on the spiritual path, as it climbs the ladder of the chakras and brings awareness. The symbol is drawn from the crown down the spine, front or back, to clear and open the channel. Some say it does activate the kundalini itself, raising the physical metabolism when the body is energetically depleted, as well as aligning the chakras. It is drawn to start many attunement processes. To activate it, one chants "Nin Giz Zida," "Serpent of Fire," or "Tibetan Serpent."

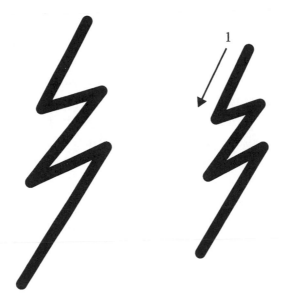

Figure 13: Grounding Symbol

Grounding Symbol

Called Raku ("ra-ku"), this lightning bolt–like symbol is also drawn from the crown to the base or feet, to ground the recipient of the attunement and separate the auras of the teacher and student. It is also used to ground a client at the end of the session. I know a teacher who teaches this symbol in Reiki One for that reason alone. Raku symbolizes completion and is used to end attunements and sessions. Previously I stated that it is used to separate the auras of the student and teacher during the attunement process. Some people only use it for that purpose, but it can also be used in the context of a healing session to separate people in an unhealthy relationship, or separate someone from their unhealthy attachments and bad habits. It doesn't necessarily end the relationship or completely end attachments or habits; it puts "distance" between the person and the object of their unhealthy connection. The symbol of Raku is like the bolt of enlightenment that Dr. Usui received on the mountaintop at the end of his quest. Although I learned it as a separate symbol, and use it as such, some feel it is a variation of the Serpent of Fire, and is attributed to Tibetan origins. The feel of the symbol and its uses are different from the Tibetan Serpent. I think the power of Raku is still being discovered.

Antahkarana

Antahkarana ("an-ta-ka-ra-na") is the last symbol taught in many Reiki traditions. The word antahkarana means "spiritual organ" in Vedic lore, perhaps referring to the mind or invisible essence. According to the teachings of author Alice Bailey, the Antahkarana indicates a column of light descending into the crown chakra and is associated with the central column connecting the chakras, called the Sushuma in the Hindu traditions. Now the word is associated with a visual symbol. This image cannot be drawn in the traditional way and is not used in the traditional attunement process, but many Reiki practitioners keep a picture of it in their healing room, or under the table. The Shamballa tradition uses it in the attunement process through visualization and chanting.

The powers attributed to this symbol are many. It is said that if you gaze at it for a short time, it will automatically connect you to your higher self, start the microcosmic orbit (which is described later in this chapter), open and cleanse all the chakras, induce a meditative state, and connect you with your guides and angels. The symbol will cleanse crystals and jewelry if they are placed on it or between two Antahkarana images. I don't feel drawn to use it often, though I do think there is a power to it. My teacher suggests from her guidance that it is only for critical emergency use. If you choose to use it, you can keep a photo of it, gaze at it, chant the name, or simply visualize it. Through psychic information, it is considered to be ancient Chinese, Atlantean, Lemurian, and of course Tibetan. A popular folk tale in the Reiki community concerns its Tibetan origin. Tibetan-tradition Reiki Masters recently brought the symbol to groups of Tibetan monks who were traveling through the United States, hoping to learn its true origin and power. When asked, the monks responded, "That's very beautiful, but we've never seen it before."

To me, the Antahkarana symbol is very reminiscent of the Celtic triskallion symbol, which is often thought of by modern pagans as a symbol of the triple goddess. Triple imagery balances the mind, body, and spirit, and also symbolizes the principles of generation, organization, and destruction. The three spirals also symbolize the three trimesters of pregnancy.

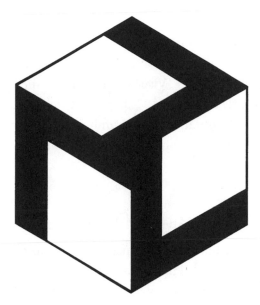

Figure 14: Antahkarana

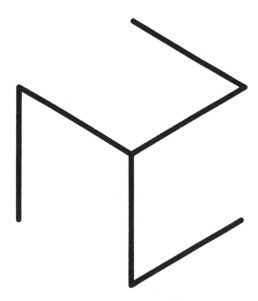

Figure 15: Triskallion

Exercise: Symbol Meditation

Choose a symbol you wish to connect with on a deeper level, from either Reiki Two or the Master level. Make sure you memorize it. Relax your mind and your body, getting into a comfortable meditative state. Visualize the symbol the best you can. Chant the name of the symbol silently or out loud. Call upon the Reiki energy to guide you. Imagine yourself going into the vibration of the symbol and be aware of your experience, whatever it may be. When done, gently return yourself from this meditative state and thank the energy of Reiki.

Passing Attunements

Passing attunements seemed like the most magickal thing to me when I got involved in Reiki. Such a mystique surrounded them. Even though I had been doing real magick for many years, you could read about real magick in most bookstores by then. But nothing was really available on Reiki, at least nothing that explained what the attunement was or how it worked. In my Reiki One class, my teacher could not or would not explain what the attunement was. All I was told was that Reiki attunes your chakras to the universal life force. Of course, I asked how, but got no answer. Many traditional Reiki teachers will not even reveal that symbols are a part of Reiki until you take level two. In the end, the attunement process turned out to be another magickal ritual.

The attunement process is an initiation. In many magickal traditions, a teacher will pass the energy of the tradition to the student through a ritual that awakens and opens the student to the energy. A greater sense of magickal power, psychic ability, and spiritual awareness is often a byproduct of the ritual.

As with all rituals, intent, energy, and symbolism are all part of the ritual. The Reiki Master basically builds up a "charge" of energy and uses it to attune the student's energy to this particular vibration. The Master and practitioner symbols are drawn in the student's aura to help direct, stabilize, and pass the energy smoothly and easily. The person passing the attunement doesn't even have to have an awareness of the energy. Anyone attuned to the Reiki Teacher level, following an attunement formula, can pass on the energy. No psychic skill is really needed.

Another Reiki teacher gave me a great analogy for the attunement process, particularly for those unfamiliar with initiation rituals. Reiki is like a frequency, and the Reiki Master is one who knows how to tune our internal radio to the frequency. The attunement process lets us tune in to the frequency whenever it is needed, raising our internal "antenna" to receive it. Each level of Reiki training raises the antenna higher and clears the static, allowing the signal to come in stronger. Even if you have only one attunement, the more you use Reiki, the more you clearly tune in and raise your antenna. You simply need the first attunement to start the process.

Some practitioners think the attunement process is like rocket science or chemistry; if you don't have the precise formula, you will mess it up and it won't work. In fact, one very conservative Reiki Master in my area has encouraged this line of thought to use fear to keep students in his tradition. Terrible consequences are given for those who are not attuned with Usui's exact formula and you are in danger of drawing on your own ki and harming yourself beyond repair. But in my experience, Reiki, like most magickal rituals, is more like cooking than chemistry. Initiation rituals have been changed. Tibetan symbols have been added. New traditions are created like new recipes, and everyone I know is just fine. Individual teachers make the process more complicated or simple to suit their own tastes and needs.

Although I'll be sharing with you the method of attunement I originally learned, I've noticed that attunements are as unique as the people getting them. Yes, I follow this basic formula, a combination of Diane Stein's and the Center for Reiki Training's methods, but I find that I tend to vary the process as I'm doing it, so each attunement is not exactly the same. For example, the time between steps may be different, or my psychic impression of it may be different. Or sometimes the symbols come out in a different order than I had planned.

Preparing for the Attunement Process

The most important thing to remember for the attunement process is intention. The techniques described here aid the energy transfer, but they are not absolutely vital. Some teachers find these two exercises pivotal, while others omit them completely. I've seen attunements work in both cases. I find them a beneficial practice for both energetic health and a great focus for the attunement ritual.

The first technique is called the Hui Yin position, and it has caused a great deal of stress among aspiring Reiki teachers. It is actually much easier to do than you might think, but it is difficult to put into words. Here is one time where I truly understand the need for a physical, in-person teacher to make sure the student understands the process, but I will nonetheless endeavor to explain it.

The Hui Yin is said to be an open circuit in the energy system. At this particular point, the line of energy is broken and can only be reconnected through intent and a muscular contraction. The muscle used is the PC muscle, which is the same muscle used when urinating. Many people are familiar with it through Kegel exercises. You can practice holding and releasing this contraction regularly, to really feel the muscle and build your stamina and coordination.

The entire circuit is not complete with just the Hui Yin position. Although most healers imagine the energy flow of the chakras as a central column, often with a double helix of two other circuits, flowing up through the center of the body or inside the spine, the particular energy circuit of this Reiki technique is different. It seemingly lies outside the body, or near the skin surface. The circuit goes up the back and spine, over the skull, down the brow and face, through the tongue, into the neck, chest, and belly, down to the groin, and back to the Hui Yin point to start again. Some visualizations of this extend the flow down the back of the legs, up the feet, and then up the front of the legs, back to the Hui Yin, then moving up the back, to create a figure-eight shape instead of a loop. But to complete the circuit, one must press the tongue to the roof of the mouth, behind the teeth, to allow the energy to flow down, while simultaneously holding the Hui Yin. The practice of flowing energy through this circuit is called the Microcosmic Orbit, sometimes abbreviated as MCO.

Exercise: Microcosmic Orbit

Contract the Hui Yin position and put the tongue to the roof of the mouth. Many people think the Hui Yin must be clenched, but a simple contraction is more than sufficient since you will be moving around during the attunement process. Simply bend forward slightly and stick your buttocks out. As you straighten, contract the buttocks slightly, along with the PC muscle. That is the amount of pressure needed with the PC muscle. You can now relax your buttocks. You can contract more, holding a tight lock, but that's up to you. In the end, I think intention is the most important part. If you can't hold the contraction, that won't prevent the energy from flowing if you will it to flow.

Once you are in position, intend to create a ball of energy near the navel. Allow it, visualize it, and it will be a reality. Hold the ball of energy as it builds in intensity. Feel it

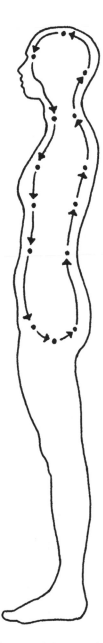

Figure 16: Microcosmic Orbit

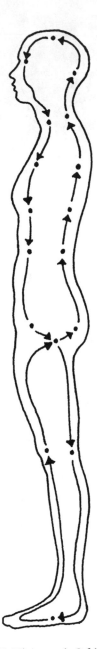

Figure 17: Microcosmic Orbit Extended

get heavier. Then drop the ball down this Microcosmic Orbit pathway. Feel it flow down to the Hui Yin, cross over, and go up the back. Feel it move up the neck and head, down the face and through the tongue. Move the ball into the throat, chest, and back to the belly. Repeat, finding a pace all your own. (As you become more comfortable with it, you can try the Figure Eight position of the extended MCO.) The ball may even feel elusive, becoming one long stream of energy. The visualization isn't as important as feeling the flow along these circuits.

Make several repetitions. You can meditate on this orbit, or let it fade from your consciousness, absorbing the energy back into your system as you release the hold on the Hui Yin and tongue.

One does not have to do Reiki to do the MCO. It predates our modern concept of Reiki, coming from Taoist practice, and is a technique to increase the health and vitality of anyone who practices it. The hold reminds me of the Muldaban, or Root Lock, of Kundalini yoga, used to raise consciousness up the spine and chakras. When the circuit is held during Reiki sessions by the Reiki practitioner, it increases the ability to channel Reiki energy and often grants the practitioner more awareness, clarity, and a sense of guidance.

The last preparatory technique for attunement is called the Violet Breath or the Dragon Breath, depending on the tradition. They are basically the same thing. The Violet Breath is a technique that helps you build up a charge of Reiki energy to transfer to the student during the attunement process. It is associated with violet, as many spiritual traditions use the color violet for transmutation. The Violet Breath aids the student in transmuting any unhealthy energy blocks that could impede the flow of Reiki. It opens the person's system to receive the attunement. You use the Hui Yin and MCO to transfer the "packet" of Reiki energy to the student. The version presented here is heavy on visualization, but if you don't see the colors, simply know they are present as needed. The feeling of connection, guidance, and healing is the most important thing in Reiki, not color. We are using the symbols of the Earth and Sky, but Reiki energy is beyond Earth and Sky. Reiki is universal and not limited to direction, but visualizing it as coming from the Earth and Sky helps our human consciousness feel connected with it. To me, visualization of the Violet Breath energies are a way to help me connect to the energy and pass an attunement. If such visualizations hinder you, disregard them and simply focus on your intention to pass a Reiki attunement.

Exercise: Violet Breath

Hold the Hui Yin position and put the tongue to the roof of the mouth. Be aware of the MCO pathway, and begin the energy flow along the pathway. Intend to connect to the Earth. Inhale and feel "blue" Earth energy of Reiki rise up from the planet and into your feet, entering the Microcosmic Orbit, turning the orbit blue. Exhale.

Intend to connect with the Sky. Inhale and feel "white" Sky energy of Reiki descend down into your crown, mixing with the blue Earth energy, creating a light blue orbit. Exhale.

Intend to connect with the stars. Inhale and feel the "red" star energy of Reiki descend into your brow, mixing with the blue and white energy, creating a violet light in the orbit. Exhale and breathe normally. Feel the energy build with the violet light.

During the attunement process, the Reiki Master visualizes the Master symbol (I use the Tibetan Master symbol) in the mouth. Some draw the symbol on the roof of their mouth. I simply visualize it and chant the symbol silently three to nine times. The violet energy and Master symbol is exhaled into the student's crown during the attunement. If you are practicing this without doing an attunement, you can blow it into the room to release the energy.

Even if you don't see color or feel the energy, simply know that it is occurring and that the Reiki is flowing through you and will allow you to transfer the energy as needed.

Passing Reiki Initiations

The training of a Reiki teacher is the training in how to pass an attunement to students, to empower them to become practitioners. Most believe that only those at the Reiki Master level have a sufficient energy level to pass the attunements, but through experimentation, other rogues have found that anyone attuned to Reiki can pass an attunement if they know the process. Attunements done by a Reiki Master simply seem to have the greatest effect on the student, and traditionally, only Reiki Masters have the knowledge of the Master symbols. Each attunement has slightly different symbols, so many feel that if you do not hold that level of attunement, then you can't pass it on. Others feel that Reiki is Reiki, and that the concept of levels is manmade, not universal. If in doubt, I suggest that you seek out an experienced Reiki teacher to receive your own attunements. That way you will receive both the energy and the help to use Reiki.

Prepare yourself by centering and grounding yourself. I prepare myself for an attunement like I would a healing session. I draw the Power symbol in the six directions, and draw all the symbols in the room and on both of my palms. I call upon my highest guidance to be with me, calling upon the Reiki energy itself to guide me and flow through me. I am only an instrument.

The student sits in a comfortable straight-backed chair, feet flat on the floor and hands in prayer position, palms together at the heart. I make sure I have enough room to walk all around the chair, since I will be doing part of the attunement from the front and part in the back. I begin by standing in front of the student. I urge them to close their eyes beforehand, but it is not mandatory, as it is in some traditions. I bow and wait for a response or returned nod of the head and begin.

Part One

I stand behind the student. I draw a double Cho Ku Rei, with the "flags" pointing in, to create the image of a doorway. I pass through the doorway into a sacred space for the Reiki attunement. I think about the Reiki and hold an intention as to what kind of attunement this is, level one, two, or Master attunement. I place my hands on the student's shoulders to make an energetic connection, allowing the Reiki to flow naturally. Through my focus, I begin the Microcosmic Orbit in my body. I inhale and draw Nin Giz Zida down the back of the student, from crown to root, through the chair back, to open the chakra system to the attunement. I exhale and chant the name of the symbol three times silently in my mind. I begin the Violet Breath in the MCO and inhale, chanting the Tibetan Master symbol, Di Ko Mio, three to nine times silently. When ready, I exhale the symbol into the crown chakra. I inhale and draw the Usui Master symbol, Di Ko Myo, above the head. I guide it down into the base of the head and blow through the crown, chanting the name of the symbol silently three times.

Gently, I reach around front and guide the student's hands up to the crown, so the fingers are pointing to the sky, the base of the palms on the crown, still together in a prayer position. I inhale and draw the following symbols for each level, chanting each name three times silently and tapping them into the fingers and hands as I chant.

Level One	Level Two	Master Level
		Di Ko Mio (Tibetan)
		Di Ko Myo (Usui)
		Nin Giz Zida
Cho Ku Rei (counterclockwise)	Cho Ku Rei (double)	Cho Ku Rei (double)
Sei He Ki (single)	Sei He Ki (double)	Sei He Ki (double)
Hon Sha Ze Sho Nen	Hon Sha Ze Sho Nen	Hon Sha Ze Sho Nen
		Raku

When all symbols are done, I exhale into the fingertips, imagining the energy moving through the hands and into the crown and body. I return the student's hands back to the heart position. I inhale and continue to part two.

Part Two

I move around to the front of the student. Ideally, one should continue to hold the Hui Yin position, but if you have to break it and reconnect when you are in the front, do what is best for you. I try to hold it. Sometimes I succeed, sometimes I don't, but it doesn't seem to change the attunement much. If you need to take a breath, do so. But usually when I'm ready to transfer the energy, I inhale deeply, draw the symbols, and exhale to release the "charge."

Once in position, I guide the student's hands down and open them like a book, palms up. I hold the bottom of the hands with my left hand, to keep them steady, and leave my right hand free to draw the following symbols over the palms, chanting their names three times each, silently, and tapping them into the palms.

Level One	Level Two	Master Level
Di Ko Mio (Tibetan)	Di Ko Mio (Tibetan)	Di Ko Mio (Tibetan)
		Di Ko Myo (Usui)
		Nin Giz Zida
Cho Ku Rei (counterclockwise)	Cho Ku Rei (double)	Cho Ku Rei (double)
Sei He Ki (single)	Sei He Ki (double)	Sei He Ki (double)
Hon Sha Ze Sho Nen	Hon Sha Ze Sho Nen	Hon Sha Ze Sho Nen
		Raku

When all the symbols are in, I tap an additional three times to close the process, and close the student's hands, still holding them, in prayer position, with my left hand. The fingertips are pointing toward me. I exhale and blow the energy into the fingertips, down the chakra column to the root, and back up to the third eye, and down to the hands again. I inhale and move to part three.

Part Three

Moving behind the student again, I ask for guidance for any final intentions, thoughts, blessings, or symbols to come through me from the divine. Sometimes I am conscious of them, and sometimes I am not, but in either case, I blow whatever is for the highest good of the student into the crown chakra. At this point, I relax my breath and inhale and exhale normally. I also release the Hui Yin and MCO.

I draw two Cho Ku Rei's at the base of the skull, asking to seal this process with the highest healing energy. I draw the Grounding symbol Raku down the back, from crown to the ground, grounding the student and making a separation of our energy fields. I chant the name of the symbol silently three times as I "push" it into the aura of the student, without necessarily touching the student.

Part Four

Coming to the front again, I sweep any remaining Reiki energy toward the student and say a final blessing, usually something like this: "We are both blessed by the gifts of Reiki. You are a Reiki Practitioner (or Master). Namaste." Namaste is generally translated to mean "the divine within me honors the divine within you." It's become a New Age welcome, blessing, and farewell, much like the pagan "Blessed be."

Any attunement is only needed once, though many in the strict Usui tradition separate the first attunement into four shorter attunements. For those uncertain about the energy transfer, the Reiki One attunement can be passed four times over one to two days, to reinforce the flow and clear the pathways. It's still a Reiki One attunement, but facilitates the perception of the energy by a timid Reiki teacher and student. It is not necessary. One attunement works sufficiently. The Reiki Two attunement can be passed twice over one or two days. The Reiki Three attunement is only necessary once, but many like to do it twice, representing the practitioner level of energy and the teaching level of energy. These are simply guidelines. Do as you feel intuitively or psychically guided.

Individuality in Attunements

Notice how I stressed in the attunement description and instruction that *I* do it a certain way. I did that because that is the attunement I learned, with a few modifications, and the one I use. Not every Reiki teacher uses it. If you become a Reiki teacher, you might learn something completely different. Remember, it is more like cooking than chemistry. Modify the recipe to suit you. Simplify the ritual as needed, or make it more intricate if you are compelled to do so. The process is not as difficult as it might seem. Memorize the steps, but if you need to review or use a "cheat sheet" when starting out, it's okay. I practiced on empty chairs for weeks, pretending to attune people, to get the hang of the mechanics of the process. In the end, let go of your doubts, and do it the best way you can.

I notice that not all Reiki traditions put the Usui Master symbol in the base of the skull, as I was taught. I later learned that in some traditions of Native American hands-on healing, the medicine person would "go to the back of the head" to retrieve their "medicine." Once they meditated on this spot, one or both of their hands would vibrate and shake, indicating that they could now do hands-on healing and have the healing medicine present. If they did not bring their consciousness into the brain stem, the healing would not take place. Perhaps this energy point is a well of healing energy, connecting us to the universal life force, regardless of tradition.

Notes on the Attunement

The following are some practical considerations that few books and teachers talk about for the attunement. I was lucky to have teacher who was not only mystical, but also very down to earth. Think about these before doing attunements if you reach the teaching level of Reiki.

Breath

You should consider putting a drop of essential oil, such as peppermint or lavender, on your tongue for your breath when blowing air at your students. At the very least, make sure you have brushed your teeth or taken a mint. It sounds silly, but you may forget to do so after you've had lunch or a snack during an earlier break. Avoid commercial perfumes since many people are allergic to them.

Chair

Make sure the chair is comfortable for the student and you can easily walk around it. Be careful of chair placement. I prefer open spaces in the room and have the student facing magnetic north. It's my personal preference, but not necessary. North is just my favorite magickal direction. I avoid seating people under beams or in corners because it disrupts the flow of energy.

Self-Treatment After the Attunement

Make sure the student does at least five minutes of a self-treatment after the attunement to ground the energy. If the student does not, headaches or an ungrounded feeling can occur.

Meditations Before the Attunement

Sometimes guided meditations help greatly in creating a deeper and richer experience for the student. They can be quick and simple, either opening up the chakras with colored light and meditating on each one, or a guided journey to meet a spirit guide or angel (see chapter 9).

Ritual Aspects

Candles, music, incense, tone, and light all play into the ritual setting and mood. Ritual helps us focus energy and intention and make the Reiki attunement a special, magickal time. Although I prefer a ritual setting, I have also done attunements in crowded hospital rooms, and they worked just as well.

Fasting

Due to Dr. Usui's fast on his mountaintop, some students like to fast before the attunement. I don't require it, particularly of my level one and two students, but my student and friend Michelle suggested for the Master level that students fast for twenty-one hours before the initiation, symbolic of Usui's twenty-one-day fast. I sometimes suggest it to people, but never make it a requirement. Everybody has different dietary needs. If you do fast, make sure to drink water, or if it seems too harsh, consider a juice fast. If in doubt, consult a qualified medical healthcare provider.

Healing Attunements

Healing attunements are done in a similar manner to traditional attunements, except the focus is in the heart or head, and no symbols are passed through the hand chakras. The activation of the hand chakras is what attunes a practitioner to share the energy through the hands. When the Reiki Master attunes a client to the Reiki energy but does not attune the hands, the recipient cannot then practice Reiki. The client receives all the healing effects of an attunement, including purging unwanted energies and an increased sense of spiritual connection, but does not have the ability to practice Reiki and does not need to take Reiki One training to use the energy effectively.

The two main ways of doing an attunement are sitting up in a chair or lying down on a table. Many practitioners use a chair because that is how they normally pass attunements. Others already have their client on a table and make it a part of the treatment process without disrupting the flow by having a client get up at any point. There are no rules to healing attunements. They are not a part of traditional Reiki. Make your own formulas and do what feels right. Here are some suggestions.

Healing Attunement in a Chair

This is more like a Reiki initiation ritual than a healing session, but it is very powerful. Do it exactly like a practitioner attunement, but have the client keep his or her hands on the lap. Blow the following symbols in through the crown and focus on them landing and centering in the heart space. I often see the energy radiating from the heart to heal the body.

Di Ko Mio (Tibetan) on the Violet Breath

Di Ko Myo (Usui)

Nin Giz Zida

Cho Ku Rei

Sei He Ki

Hon Sha Ze Sho Nen

Raku

Come around to the front of the client and draw the same sequence of symbols into the heart chakra. Blow from the heart chakra, to the root, to the third eye, and back to the heart. Go around to the back and give a silent blessing, such as "You are completely healed," releasing the Hui Yin and MCO. Go around to the front and give a final blessing, such as "We are both blessed by the gifts of Reiki. Namaste."

Healing Attunement on a Table

There are two ways this can be done, either separately or together:

1) While at the client's head, either sitting or standing, visualize the crown chakra opening. Use the Violet Breath and MCO to blow the sequence of symbols in, as a group or individually, through the crown and into the heart. Or simply visualize the symbols entering the crown when you draw them.

2) With your hands on the heart position, contract the Hui Yin and do the MCO. Chant silently and visualize the sequence of symbols entering the heart chakra, as just described in the instructions for the healing attunement in a chair.

You do not have to use breath work unless you want to do so. You can chant out loud or silently. You can draw the symbols or simply visualize them. You make the call. In any healing attunement, always have the intention that "this healing attunement is for your highest good." Have no judgment or expectations. All Reiki practitioners can use healing attunements, using the symbols they know, regardless of their level of training. Healing attunements are a creative way of using the symbols in a session.

Teaching Tips for Reiki Masters

Although we call the Reiki Master level of training "teacher training," no one can teach you to truly be a teacher. I have found experience and desire to be the best teachers, and I have learned as much from my "failures" as my successes. Most people become Reiki Masters without a desire to teach formally, though sooner or later, someone will probably ask you to teach them. I highly suggest passing on both the energy and the knowledge to use it. Teaching Reiki has been one of the most rewarding experiences in my life, and I actually prefer teaching Reiki to doing Reiki sessions. I would rather empower people than have them come to me when they need help.

If you decide to teach, discover the style that best suits you and your life and prepare accordingly. Most teach informally, attuning family, friends, and clients in a relaxed, demonstrative style and through personal stories. A semiformal practice is structured more like a class, but you are not necessarily out in the world advertising your services as a teacher and putting on demonstrations, clinics, and classes at metaphysical and holistic stores. If you do decide to practice Reiki as a full- or part-time profession, you must have the necessary experience to teach properly, perhaps starting out in a less formal style, as well as the necessary materials, including teaching manuals and certificates. You can use the first few chapters of this book as an introductory textbook or manual from which to build your class foundation, particularly if you have magickally oriented students, rather than those with a more medical focus.

Keep the following points in mind as well, when designing your classes.

Class Size

If you are more comfortable teaching one-on-one classes, then do so. If you prefer larger groups, then do that. Group energy can be wonderfully inspiring, but doing a large number of attunements can be tiring. Individual classes can be relaxed or very intense, depending on the student.

Schedules

Some teachers prefer to set teaching schedules and project for class registration, while others schedule classes as people inquire. Either way is fine. If you need to set dates and to devote yourself to teaching, instead of filling the time with other events and responsibilities, set monthly dates. After teaching for a year, you will have a good idea of how to plan your schedule.

Be Prepared

Have an outline of what you plan on teaching so you don't get lost, but be flexible enough to let the course go with the flow of questions. Don't be afraid to read something out of your notes. Meditations can be read, or some teachers use prerecorded meditations.

Share

Share personal stories, feelings, and memories of Reiki, your own classes, sessions, and your own healing journey. Anyone can read a manual on Reiki, but people will be drawn to your own stories and experiences and how they can relate. That is why I require a six-month waiting period between level two and the Master level, for students to start gathering their stories. Many people like to hear what could happen when working on someone. They like to hear how you handled situations, and now, older and wiser, how you would handle them again. Share mistakes along with successes, so others can learn from your early fumblings. So many people get involved with Reiki for their own healing, and knowing that you, the teacher, are experiencing healing takes you from the level of honored Reiki Master to that of a normal human being, which is what a Reiki Master is. As a normal, healing, and fallible person, students can identify with you better and possibly aspire to become Reiki Masters themselves.

Let Others Share

Although you, the teacher, are the primary focus, allow others to share their experiences and make the group interactive. People like to be "talked to" and, even more, "talked with," as opposed to "talked at." I start my classes with introductions and give everyone a chance to say why they are at Reiki class. When we do meditations, exercises, or attunements, there is a chance to share experiences with others, so no one is wondering "Was my experience weird?" I encourage students to ask questions, and I do not always have to be the one to answer them. Sometimes leading people to the answers rather than simply answering them is the best way. They know already and will feel that much more confident when confronted with a question on their own. Beware of students who want to monopolize the floor and gently urge them to let others have their turn. In these difficult situations, you can turn to the Native American tradition of the talking stick. Designate a stick or other object as a symbol, and whoever holds it can talk, and whoever doesn't have it must be silent. As the teacher, you can interrupt if absolutely necessary to keep the class moving.

Take Lots of Breaks

Breaks are as much for you as for your students. You need time to relax and gather yourself, and they will appreciate the time to absorb the knowledge and information. Plan an appropriate lunch time if your class runs that long. Do not try to cook for the class and teach. Buy or prepare food in advance. Have students bring a lunch or have resources nearby where students can dine. Teaching is strenuous enough without adding any additional responsibilities.

Drink Lots of Water

Being sufficiently hydrated helps you pass the Reiki energy during classes and in sessions. Drinking lots of water also soothes the throat. If you are not used to talking for extended periods of time, make tea or take cough drops. Encourage your students to drink a lot of water, too, to help their personal cleansing.

Dress Comfortably

Nothing is worse than feeling uncomfortable for a five- to eight-hour class when you can't go home and change.

Your Own Training

Use the Reiki classes you took and the experiences you had as a guide. If you liked the experience, try to recreate it and build upon it. If you didn't, then try to make the class what you would enjoy.

Observe Other Teachers

Observe not only Reiki Masters, but the teachers of any class you take. From college accounting to yoga to auto mechanics, information is imparted many ways. See what other teachers do as part of their style and incorporate the things you like into your own. I have incorporated wonderful techniques from art, music, and yoga teachers along with my Reiki Master's style. We are all influenced by our teachers, like musicians are influenced by the music they listen to and play.

Ask for Higher Guidance

Ask the Reiki energy and Reiki guides to teach through you (see chapter 9). Surprisingly, the words will be there even if you did not know the answers yourself. Be open to intuition and guidance.

Know Your Limits

Most Reiki teachers cannot teach every day, six days a week. The energy is simply too intense. Take time off and rest when needed.

Don't Believe Your Own Press

When in a role that helps others with their healing, we often become the center of attention and focus with bright blessings and praise. It is a wonderful feeling to have others validate your contribution. When enough people see you through rose-colored glasses, telling you that you are a wonderful spiritual being, a "master teacher," a "guide," or an "enlightened" being, it is easy to forget that you are human too. You have all the benefits and limitations of being in a human body in the physical plane. You are still here to develop and grow. Helping others is a part of the process. Do not think just because you are a healer that you are no longer learning or growing on this plane. Keep grounded, centered, and down to earth with people. Give everyone the attention they need, but realize that we are all similar, seeking similar things and learning similar lessons. Remember how this all felt to you when it was brand new, be it Reiki, psychic abilities, or any type of spiritual awakening.

Relax and Have Fun

If you aren't having fun, then chances are no one else is, so relax. Lighten up. Tell a joke. Healing classes should be happy, not frightening or painful.

The Business of Reiki

If you choose to do Reiki in a professional context, be it as a practitioner or a teacher, it has to be run like a business. Some of the more modern and down-to-earth tales show Dr. Usui not as a teacher, but a businessman who applied his skills to bring Reiki to more people. In a system that asks for an exchange, making a business of this service is in no way dishonorable. Many people feel that if something is spiritual, it shouldn't have to cost anything. But to me, everything is spiritual. Food, clothing, art, music, ritual tools, herbs, toys, medicine—they are all sacred and have their place in my life. Reiki is just as valuable to some people, and as practitioners we must be honored for our time and service. Establishing a full-time practice where you are readily available to the public can be a big risk, both financially and personally, so you must be compensated for your time and effort.

Not everyone is successful doing Reiki, or any metaphysical discipline, full-time. Some claim that all these metaphysicians, psychics, mediums, and gurus are seeking to get rich quick, but let me assure you, it is not a quick and easy road to success. Being an alternative modality, there is no guarantee that even with education, there will be a desire for the service in your area. If you hope to be successful at Reiki on this level, you must treat it like a business, with a business plan, advertising and promotional materials, accounting, marketing and so on, like any other enterprise. Study information on starting a business or building a home business. Many of the same principles will apply, but in this case, you will have the power of the universal life force flowing through you unencumbered, and guiding you, if you choose to listen.

Healing Fear

Becoming a Reiki Master is ultimately about claiming your full power to actively heal yourself and help others heal. As with any spiritual practice, with Reiki, we are forced to confront our fears, our darker self and shadow self. These are the things that are repressed in us, but contain valuable lessons for our own practice if we learn to accept and love them. Healing the shadow to claim personal power is a key component of many magickal traditions, from shamanism to witchcraft.

We all create our own reality. You've probably heard that many times. So what happens when you are experiencing a reality you don't want? Why would you create pain or suffering? If the conscious you is not creating your reality, the repressed and often detached part of you is creating the reality in an effort to get attention. Your shadow creates the shadow reality. Part of healing is bringing all disconnected and lost aspects of the self back into the fold. Actively healing our shadow and our seed fears, the fears we allow to grow into issues that hinder our healing process, is the first job of the Reiki Master.

One of the most common concerns of newly initiated Reiki Masters is the decision not to teach or attune others because of fear: fear they will not do a good job, fear the attunement will not work, or ultimately fear of claiming these new aspects of their power. Many claim that one is not a Reiki teacher with the third attunement; one is only a Reiki teacher after passing at least one attunement. I encourage all of my Master students to go home and attune someone, anyone, before the week is over, just to get over the fear. At this point, the attunement seems, to some, a monumental task, one that will never be memorized or internalized, so why bother? Fear of your own power and abilities, even the power to pass attunements and do Reiki, is part of your shadow self. As a Reiki Master, it is your job to acknowledge your fears and actively work on healing them.

Teaching and passing attunements are two of the most empowering parts of the Reiki Master process. An introspective practice, such as journaling, meditation, prayer, shamanism, or any other spiritual practice, is necessary to identify and face these aspects of the self. If you are not part of a spiritual tradition, find the elements of traditions that call to you and start creating your own. Study aspects of magick and mysticism to learn about your shadow in a deep and personal way. Healing the shadow is a lifelong process. Acknowledge and heal each layer of the shadow as it surfaces. It is your responsibility to heal this fear, but you should get help through a facilitator when you need it. Just because you are a Reiki Master does not mean you can't accept help from other healers, including other Reiki practitioners. Be open to healing facilitation for yourself. If you help others heal themselves, let others help you heal.

Another Beginning

In the end, many people see the Reiki Master level as the ultimate level. To those who view martial arts such as karate or kung fu from the outside, earning a black belt seems like the ultimate degree of mastery. But any practitioner knows that such achievements are only the first step on the real path. I think Reiki is the same way, I suggest that all students think about completing the Master level, even if they have no desire to teach or practice formally. I originally completed my Master training for myself. If it served others, that was great, but I needed to have the sense of completeness for myself, to really put it to use in my life. It wasn't until I achieved this level that Reiki became such a vast part of my life. Remember, this is only the first step in a grander adventure. When you receive an initiation, even if it is the final initiation of a tradition, it is another beginning. To initiate means to begin, and as your students begin a path, you too will be transformed, beginning again and again with them.

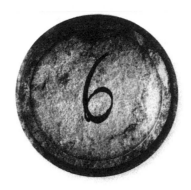

Beyond Usui: New Traditions of Reiki

Although each level of Reiki is complete in and of itself, and the Master teacher level is the culmination of all levels, many people leave this training with a sense of incompleteness. I had a great experience with my training and felt confident to be a Reiki teacher, but I felt like something was missing too.

All the talk of the ancient traditions of Reiki makes me wonder if we have the full picture. Secret histories, secret symbols, and new inspired and channeled information have me wondering what are the roots of Reiki, and how can I get back to them? Did Usui only figure out half the formula? Was there more he didn't find or understand before going down the mountain to put it into action? Even if he had the whole formula, why am I not capable of the same miracles he was capable of?

The first and most obvious answer is that the Reiki story has grown in mythic proportions and that Usui did not physically accomplish these things. The second answer is that perhaps he had the whole formula, but didn't pass it on, or one of his students decided not to pass it on. Did Takata receive the complete teachings? She was both a woman and a foreigner, so perhaps she was not accepted completely, and thus she passed an incomplete teaching. We just don't know, and the endless speculation can make it difficult to make peace.

Even before I heard about these theories, I felt like there was something missing to Reiki, something unrevealed. During all of my attunements, I saw light form into strange geometrical shapes—symbols—but they were unlike the symbols I learned in the tradition. I was told by other teachers that they were personal symbols, for my own healing, not to be used on others. But I found myself guided to use them in my work with clients.

Soon I learned about expanded forms of Reiki, which promised to teach the lost symbols and lost information about this ancient healing art, moving beyond the Usui training into the realms of ancient Egypt or Atlantis. I was interested in learning more, and found there was a large group of variant Reiki traditions. None were accepted by the Reiki Alliance, but each had something special to offer. Some were complete traditions, while others were expansions or additions to the Usui or Usui Tibetan traditions.

Very little has been written about these traditions in the public record, besides the vast arena of the Internet. Written information comes from manuals in these traditions, as well as posts and personal anecdotes from students and teachers. As we move further and further away from traditional Usui Reiki, the information becomes less cohesive and more personal. Two people could have learned the same tradition, with the same name, but learned very different things, depending on the teacher. Such variety is wonderful, but makes it hard to give thorough descriptions, since the practice changes with each practitioner's line of teaching. The material cannot be found in any mainstream published book, but rather in hand-copied, reworked manuals, if printed at all. There are conflicts in trainings and histories, but they all expand upon the standard Usui material.

Modern Reiki Traditions

Here are some of the modern traditions of Reiki that have added much to my modern, magickal understanding of the healing art. Their individuality, variety, and sacred geometry have inspired me to bring more individuality to my own practice of healing.

Usui Shiki Ryoho

This is the Usui tradition of Hayashi and Takata. This is the best-known form of Reiki in the West.

Usui Reiki Ryoho

This is the tradition of Reiki practiced in Japan. There is greater emphasis on particular meditation techniques and empowerment rituals, rather than symbols and the more commonly known Reiki attunement process. There are a variety of non-Takata traditions in Japan as well, often with a strong Buddhist foundation.

Usui Tibetan Reiki

This is an addition to the traditional Hayashi-Takata form of Reiki, incorporating "Tibetan" symbols into the system and claiming that Reiki has origins in Tibet. The American Arthur Robertson, a student of one of Mrs. Takata's Master students, Iris Ishikuro, was reportedly the first to add the material to Reiki, creating a style called Raku Kei Reiki. Later, it became the basis of what is known now as the Usui Tibetan tradition. The belief that Reiki originated in Tibet has been popularized by many teachers, although there is little hard evidence of it.

The Radiance Technique®

Barbara Ray is one of the Reiki Masters trained by Takata. After Takata's passing, Ray claimed that Takata had given her "all" the attunements in a six-level (some say seven-level) system. Initially calling it Real Reiki®, she later renamed it the Radiance Technique®.

Seichim

Patrick Zeigler is considered the founder of the traditions called Seichim, though a variety of spellings exist. Seichim is the vital life force component of the soul in Egyptian mysticism, considered to be the equivalent of prana, rauch, or ki in other systems. Zeigler spent time in the Middle East in 1979 to 1980, including spending a night in the Great Pyramid of Giza, where he received a spontaneous initiation. He experienced an unusual, mystical connection to what would later by called the Seichim energy. After his pyramid experience, he spent time studying with a Sufi sheikh. After his journeys in the

East, he returned to the United States and received Reiki training from Barbara Ray. He used the Reiki attunement process and divine guidance to transfer the Seichim energy to others. The Sufis he had studied with danced in an infinity pattern, so the infinity symbol, rather than the spiral, plays a strong role in this tradition.

Later, Zeigler worked with Christine Gerber, who chaneleled a spirit guide that named the Seichim energy and initially guided its use. Zeigler collaborated with many others in the creation of this system, bringing a variety of styles, traditions, and symbols under the Seichim umbrella. Some of these Seichim traditions involved a form of Egyptian mythology and mysticism, including Isis Seichim, relating to the Egyptian goddess Isis, and also Sekhemet Seichim and Sekhem, both involving the lion goddess Sekhmet. Angel Seichim is a tradition that uses the Judeo-Christian archangels in the healing process. The most common system is the seven-facet Seichim, originated by Phoenix Summerfield, one of the early practitioners involved in the birth of Seichim with Zeigler. Patrick now teaches SKHM, simplifying the energy and focusing on a guided meditation to connect to the energy, rather than symbol attunements. Diane Ruth Shewmaker has continued to pioneer new practices in the tradition, and her book *All Love: A Guidebook for Healing with Sekhem-Seichim-Reiki and SKHM* is an excellent resource for all those interested in this tradition.

Tera Mai™ Reiki and Tera Mai Seichim™

These are traditions founded by Kathleen Milner, author of *Reiki & Other Rays of Touch Healing* and *Tera: My Journey Home*. While at a Whole Life Expo in 1991, Kathleen was introduced to Seichim and later was guided to incorporate some of this new material and energy with symbols from other sources to create a new system of Reiki. Milner has divided the energy into four elemental rays, for Earth, Water, Air, and Fire, naming each elemental ray Reiki, Sophie-El, Arcangelic, and Sakarra, respectively. She believes more traditional Seichim to be a mix of Reiki and Sakarra, or Earth and Fire.

Karuna® Reiki, Maha Karuna, and Karuna Ki

William Rand, founder of the International Center for Reiki Training, was using the same symbols that Kathleen Milner used in her tradition, but was not using the same system. Rand states that he did not intend to create a system of Reiki, but he, along with other Reiki Masters, began to experiment with these nontraditional symbols. Under spiritual guidance, he created the attunement process and system now called Karuna®

Reiki, which uses nine additional symbols and is usually taught as an update to traditional Usui Tibetan Reiki. Karuna means "compassion," and the system is often taught in association with concepts such as ascended spiritual masters, celestial beings, chanting, toning, and crystals, creating a more intricate healing system. The tradition spread, but after Rand trademarked it and set certain specific standards, many independent Reiki Masters began calling it Maha Karuna, meaning "much compassion," or Karuna Ki, "compassion energy," among other various names.

In his more traditional Reiki training, Rand suggests, via the clairvoyant Michelle Griffith, that Reiki originated in ancient Lemuria over 100,000 years ago. Lemuria is considered to be the first place where humanity incarnated, and as the Lemurian civilization progressed, the inhabitants fell from a more spiritual state into selfish emotions. A "Great Being," an aspect of the Holy Spirit, incarnated, giving the Lemurians the symbols and attunement process to reconnect with the divine. With the sinking of Lemuria, Reiki was lost, but the Great Being reincarnated two other times, once in Atlantis, where Reiki was used until Atlantis' destruction, and then later in Egypt.

Shamballa Reiki or Shamballa Multidimensional Healing

The system originally known as Shamballa Reiki was channeled by John Armitage, also known by the spiritual name Hari Das Melchizedek. He channeled the information from the ascended master referred to as St. Germain as an upgrade, or expansion, of the traditional Usui energy of Reiki. Shamballa is said to be a reclaiming of the original system, dawning at the end of Atlantis. It was originally used to help spiritually evolve certain segments of the Atlantean community, using attunements with twenty-two Master symbols. Healing ability was simply a byproduct of the increased energy and spiritual vibration. In a previous incarnation, St. Germain was the Atlantean High Priest who received this system of initiation.

Before the destruction of Atlantis, he visited the Eastern world and shared portions of the system to see what people would do with it. He feared its abuse and did not reveal the rest, allowing some of the symbols to be recorded into the Eastern scriptures. Later, Dr. Usui discovered them. St. Germain, now an ascended being after his life as a European alchemist, guided the reconstruction of Reiki, making sure it has "safeguards" and the energy cannot be used for harm.

Through St. Germain, Hari Das expanded the system further. Through a system of four levels—two practitioner levels, Master-Healer, and Master-Teacher—one is attuned to 352 symbols, representing the "352 levels back to the Divine." One doesn't memorize all these symbols. The healer simply "receives" the ones needed intuitively, consciously or unconsciously. Personally, I think there are more than 352 symbols, but the number represents symbolic energy, and practitioners receive their interpretations of the symbols as needed.

The Shamballa system is also said to contain three energies, making it unique from Reiki. The first is the original expansion of Reiki, called the Shamballa energy. Shamballa symbolizes the collective consciousness of the ascended masters, named after the mythic enlightened city of the East, and conceptualized as a great faceted crystal, where each face is the likeness of a master, but all are in union. One point is at the deepest levels of reality, and one point touches the highest levels of reality. The second energy is called the Mahatma, the Avatar of Synthesis. Described as either a white light or a mix of metallic gold and silver light with a shining glimmer of violet mixed in, Mahatma was said to be "grounded" into the world during the Harmonic Convergence in 1987 and available to anyone, with or without an attunement. It brings all oppositions into harmony. Lastly is the energy of Christ Light, not specific to Christianity, but representing the energy of the next "level of consciousness" of unconditional love, what many refer to as Christ consciousness in the New Age world. Later Shamballa was expanded to include initiations into the "twelve dimensions" of healing.

Shamballa Reiki is a collection of many ideas that are popular in the New Age community, but remains untrademarked as of this writing, and gives much flexibility to teachers. Some teach it as an update to traditional Reiki. When I completed it as an update, my entire practice changed from injury-related work to deep emotional healing. Some say the energy of Shamballa is faster than Reiki, giving you more time to talk with the client. Most teach it as a complete system and not as an update. Many combine crystals, angels, aliens, and channeling with it, while others keep it down to earth and simple. Best of all, a Fourth Degree Shamballa Master-Teacher is attuned to all 352 symbols, and many believe that these symbols include all the other symbols of all the other Reiki-related traditions. After receiving my fourth Shamballa attunement, I felt free to explore other Reiki-related symbols without necessarily being specifically attuned to that symbol or the tradition where it originated. I felt the Shamballa energy contained them all, so I didn't feel the need to go out and continually get attuned with new symbols. Despite some of my initial misgivings about the training and philosophy, the process gave me the energy to complement and complete my own Reiki training.

Shamanic Reiki

Shamanic Reiki is not a specific tradition, but a general trend that many Reiki practitioners and teachers have been exploring. It combines elements of core shamanism, including drumming, ceremony, trance work, spirit work, animal and plant spirit healing, ancestor reverence, shamanic "psychic" surgery, and guided imagery, with Reiki. Some use shamanism as a complement before or after Reiki, or use Reiki as a part of their shamanic practice. Traditionalists often feel that the two systems are incompatible, but I find they are a magickal partnership that brings wonderful healing to others.

Chaos Reiki

Chaos Reiki is another nonspecific tradition. Practitioners of it combine the concepts and attitude of a revolutionary form of ceremonial magick, called Chaos magick, with Reiki. They use Reiki not just for healing, but also to create all sorts of change and ritual. To the Chaos magician, nothing is off-limits, including the Reiki symbols. I was a member of a short-lived Internet mailing list on Chaos Reiki, and in many ways this book is inspired by that group.

Johrei® Reiki (Vajra® Reiki)

This system fuses the spiritual practice of Johrei® with Reiki. Johrei means "white light" and was founded by Mokichi Okada, a contemporary of Usui. Johrei uses a ritual somewhat similar to the earliest versions of the attunement process to empower its followers. Johrei® Reiki, using the Johrei white-light symbols, developed out of Raku Kei Reiki. The name of the Reiki tradition was changed to Vajra® Reiki. Although there may be some similarities between Johrei® and Reiki, the two are really different traditions.

Magnified Healing®

The healing technique known as Magnified Healing® is not a Reiki tradition, but shares many similarities. Brought to the general public by Kathryn Anderson and Gisele King, the original material was said to have been introduced by a "physical soul embodiment" of the ascended master Kwan Yin (sometimes spelled Quan Yin). Some view her as a goddess of mercy, compassion, and healing. The healing technique is said to heal individuals and the Earth, release karma, and help humanity ascend to a higher level of consciousness. Like Reiki, it uses an initiation process, but also has a "Magnified Healing Celebration" ceremony for many participants. Many involved in Reiki find their way to magnified healing.

Magnified Healing® is rooted in the belief system of ascension and the ascended masters. This branch of ascension-related healing is focused more on the feminine aspects of the divine, working through Quan Yin and the Shekinah. In this system, the Shekinah is defined as the Presence of God through the feminine aspect of the Holy Spirit. The divine is often referred to as The God Most High® of the universe.

Blue Star Reiki

The founder of this tradition, John Williams, a South African Reiki Master, originally called it Blue Star Celestial Energy, which he channeled from his spirit guide starting in 1995. The energy is said to bridge the gap between God and man via the Rainbow Bridge, and the knowledge of this system is said to have come from a source in an Ancient Egyptian Mystery School. Its aim is spiritual growth rather than immediate healing. William's student Gary Jirauch changed the system and renamed it Blue Star Reiki. Interestingly enough, there is a form of Wicca called Blue Star Wicca, though the two are not related.

Wei Chi Tibetan™ Reiki

This form of Reiki was received by Kevin Ross Emery and Thomas Hensel from an ancient monk named Wei Chi. Wei Chi lived over 5,000 years ago, and he and his brothers created the original system we now call Reiki. This tradition teaches Reiki the way it was done in Wei Chi's day, using not simply the laying on of hands, but also what we would now consider a form of intuitive medical diagnosis and mental/emotional/spiritual diagnosis, going beyond the simple scanning technique of many Reiki traditions. The practitioner opens up a dialogue with the client, discussing the process of becoming imbalanced and helping the client actively participate in the healing process. The process is more active than passive, distinguishing it from some forms of traditional Reiki being practiced in the West. Together, Kevin, Thomas, and the spirit of Wei Chi wrote *The Lost Steps of Reiki: The Channeled Teachings of Wei Chi.*

As you can see, the traditions of Reiki are multiplying, again and again, like a field of wild flowers, each with an exciting new shape and form. Some are rooted in spiritual traditions, particularly the Eastern traditions of Buddhism and Hinduism, and many more come from channeled inspiration. Just as it would be difficult to categorize an entire field of flowers, the task of differentiating all the traditions of Reiki is just as complex. This is a short list of those traditions with which I am most familiar, but by no means is it complete. I'm sure many more will appear in the time it takes me to write this book and for it to reach the bookstore.

The most important thing I've gleaned from this information is that all the traditions work. Everyone has a different take, but with love and guidance, they can all be healing and beneficial. I encourage people to find their own Reiki gifts and permutations, once they have a solid background and understanding of the fundamentals. I'm an eclectic witch who practices eclectic magick. I am an eclectic Reiki Master, and have the same philosophy for my students. Don't learn my tradition of Reiki—create your own. And then, with a strong understanding of the history, including what is and isn't traditional, share your tradition with others.

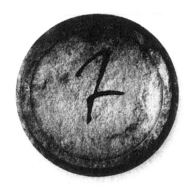

New Reiki Symbols

The "new" symbols of Reiki come from a variety of sources, such as the modern Reiki traditions discussed in chapter 6. Many claim these symbols are actually ancient, though, with a few exceptions, no ancient records of them exist. Most are inspired from a higher wisdom, through a process many people call channeling. When possible, I have listed where the symbol originates from, and in what traditions it is used, but due to the fact that the information has been passed through word of mouth, such lists are never complete. Ultimately, they all come from the same origin—the divine.

Reiki practitioners often receive symbols during attunements or sessions. To me, the process of sacred geometry seems inherent in the various energy rays of Reiki used in healing and magick. Before being involved in Reiki, I found magickal symbols to be particularly powerful forms of healing and spell casting. I used runes, seals, ogham, and other stylized sigils to create balance and change, so the Reiki symbols were a natural extension of this for me. No one really told me about the possibility of receiving symbols during the attunement, so my Reiki Two attunement was surprising.

Fear surrounds the use of new symbols for so many traditional practitioners. Personally, I think the fear stems from fear of empowerment. Reiki has been taught in a very traditional way, with tried-and-true symbols. The attitude is, if it's not broken, don't fix it. Don't add to it. Don't change it in anyway. I can understand the sentiment, but anything that doesn't grow and evolve will eventually wither away and die, because it doesn't suit the needs and temperament of those it is there to serve. The time of strict dogma, adhering to the old ways simply because that is the way it's done, is over.

Traditionalists feel the symbols are not really Reiki symbols and do not have the inherent safeguards of the traditional symbols built into them. Modernists feel that the symbols are being empowered by Reiki energy when used with Reiki, and have the same effects and safeguards as the traditional symbols.

In either case, with either belief, my answer is the same: Use your own intuition. If you are drawn to use a symbol, and it feels intuitively correct for you to use it, then use it. If a symbol doesn't feel correct to you, then don't use it. If you are not called to use symbols in your healing and magick, then don't. If you are drawn to use all the symbols, then do so.

When in doubt, simply state your intention to connect with your vision of the divine. Ask for guidance. If you are going to use a new symbol, ask that it be placed under the guidance and protection of a spirit guide, ascended master, deity, angel, or saint, so that it may be used in accord with the Reiki energy and principles, causing no harm and bring only healing, balanced, healthy energy.

The answers are so simple when we choose to view them as simple, and ask for help when we have a question or problem. Use your own intuition and guidance with the following symbols.

Zonar

Zonar is one of the most popular modern Reiki symbols, used in Tera Mai™ Reiki, Karuna® Reiki, and Shamballa Reiki. These traditions state that Zonar is used for healing issues of a "multidimensional nature" when the imbalance cannot be easily explained or understood. It is used for healing past-life issues, often along with Hon Sha Ze Sho Nen. The two can be used to heal the past trauma from this life too, particularly concerning repressed abuse issues. It also promotes deep emotional healing when undergoing an emotional release, acting as a "spiritual anesthetic" to allow the energy to be released without overwhelming the client. Zonar releases fear, hate, anger, and trauma on the cellular level. Many holistic practitioners feel that people hold such emotions on the physical, cellular plane and use a variety of techniques to release this trauma. Zonar is one powerful technique for this work. Those who work with angelic energies state that

Archangel Gabriel works with this symbol, to heal karma and to receive guidance with life questions.

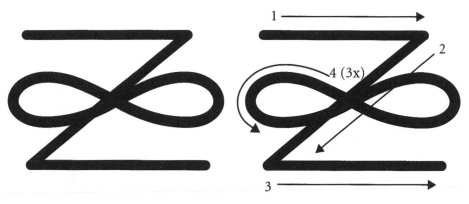

Figure 18: Zonar

Harth

Those who use Harth say it means love, truth, beauty, harmony, and balance, all the highest aspects of the divine manifest in each of us. Use it to heal the heart on all levels, to create compassion, heal unhealthy relationships, and break addictions and escapist tendencies. It brings love to those who do not see or feel love in the world, or feel buried by the burdens of the world. Harth opens one to heartfelt creativity and to spirit guides who come in love. Harth is another symbol that transforms into a temple, like a pyramid, when meditated upon. In this temple, you can receive healing and speak to guides. I have drawn Harth before a session and envisioned it expanding into a room-sized pyramid around myself and the client, to amplify the healing space and create a zone of sacred space. The apex of the pyramid acts like a vacuum, sucking up all unwanted energies released in the session. Harth is used in the Tera Mai™ Reiki and Karuna® Reiki traditions.

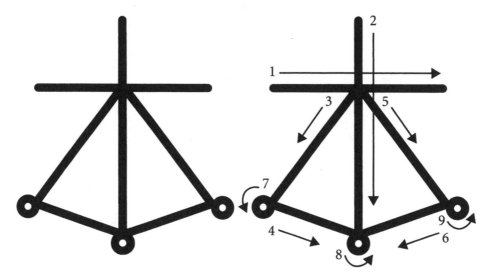

Figure 19: Harth

Halu

The symbol of Halu is a magnification of Zonar, as demonstrated by the similar shapes. Like Zonar, the infinity loop moves the healing beyond space and time, but the balanced point channels healing energy to all levels more effectively. When I have meditated upon it, Halu becomes three-dimensional and forms a structure similar to a healing temple, with the light of the universe focused through its point. Halu can be used after Zonar. This energy is used to clear unwanted thoughtforms, emotional patterns, and subconscious programs we have created or accepted from others. Halu helps us get unstuck and move out of illusion. During psychic surgery techniques (see chapter 10), use Halu to break apart the energy forms that lie at the root of illness. Like Zonar, Halu heals past abuse issues, particularly those concerning repressed sexual abuse. Halu also heals the shadow self, the part of us we have not accepted and loved. Halu is also used in the Tera Mai™ Reiki and Karuna® Reiki traditions.

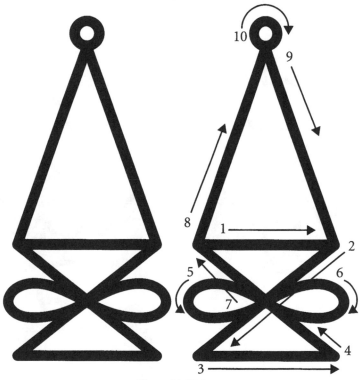

Figure 20: Halu

Mara/Rama

Mara was one of the first Reiki symbols I saw and didn't like. I like symmetry in my symbols, and when I saw it, it just seemed "off" to me. That was until I meditated on it. In three-dimensional form, it became the energy lines of the earth, with a vortex of energy in the center, like a sacred site. The five loops represent the five elements, and the two lines are the energies of male and female from the creator. Mara is a symbol of being fully present and grounded in the world. Use it on those who feel the world, or the body, is too painful or traumatic, especially at the end of a session. Mara opens the energy system and grounds, opening the feet chakras and draining unwanted energy into the earth to transmute it. Mara is used magickally to manifest in the world, empowering goal lists and wishes. Kathleen Milner calls this symbol Mara, and William Rand teaches it as Rama. I personally call it Mara when I am intuitively called to draw a clockwise spiral, and Rama when I do a counterclockwise spiral. I prefer clockwise Mara. In either case, the syllables themselves mean Ma—mother and Ra—father, so it depends on where your personal spiritual emphasis is.

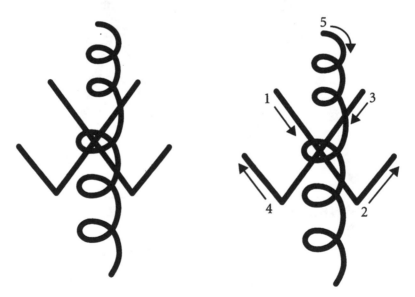

Figure 21: Mara

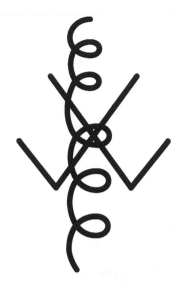

Figure 22: Rama

Gnosa

The root word of Gnosa (pronounced "no-sa," the *G* is silent) is gnosis, meaning the secret knowledge that comes from a meditative state that connects one to the divine. Use Gnosa to connect with your higher divinity. It also has a mental flair to it, used for learning new information, concepts, philosophies, and symbols. Gnosa improves communication, internally and externally, with other people in spoken, written, and artistic forms. Gnosa is a symbol for artists, musicians, and writers. The nervous system, as the great internal communicator, is healed with Gnosa.

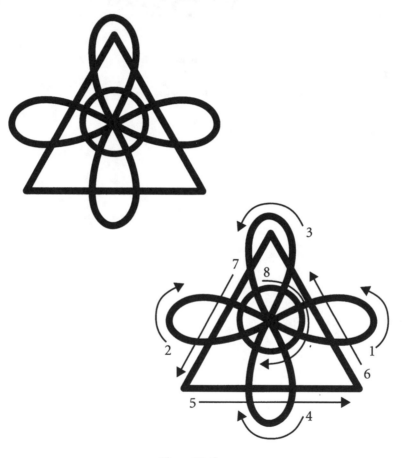

Figure 23: Gnosa

Iava

Iava (pronounced "ee-ah-vah") is used as a symbol of Earth healing and connecting with the Earth. Iava connects the user with the nature spirits and devas of a land. Symbolically, the first three spirals represent a triple goddess energy—maiden, mother, and crone—while the four loops on the "back" of the symbol are the four elements of Earth, Fire, Air, and Water. Some traditions claim that this symbol is used only for earth healing, and if used during a session on a person, it will cause harm, but I have found that to be nonsense. In people, Iava heals relationships with others, helping us claim our sovereignty and personal power in co-dependent or otherwise unhealthy relationships. This symbol is credited to Catherine Mills Bellamont of Ireland.

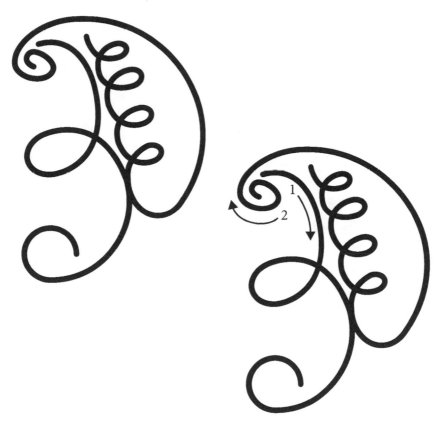

Figure 24: Iava

Kriya

Kriya is the double Cho Ku Rei, used much like the Power symbol. I use it to create a sacred space during attunements and to seal and protect a space before a session or attunement. Kriya is another earthy symbol, used for grounding, and grounding our sense of sacred in our body and physical world. It helps us focus on practical wisdom. In Kundalini yoga, the word Kriya refers to a group of exercises done over a period of forty days to manifest tangible change in the practitioner. Magickally, Kriya is used to manifest tangible results. I must admit, however, that I usually chant Cho Ku Rei with this symbol, not Kriya. Both work.

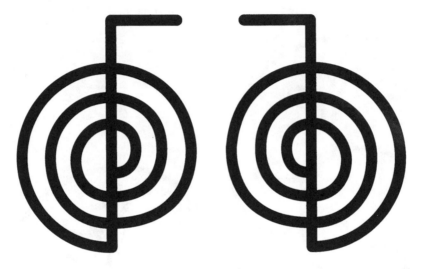

Figure 25: Kriya

Shanti

Shanti is a symbol named after a chant for peace. Chanting or drawing this symbol brings peace, healing any disturbance or restlessness by evoking a sense of inner peace. Shanti encourages us to let go of what we cannot control, being peaceful in the present. Shanti heals fear, insomnia, and chronic fatigue, and gently opens the chakras and brings clear psychic vision. It heals past traumas as well. Shanti is credited to Pat Courtney of Milwaukee, WI.

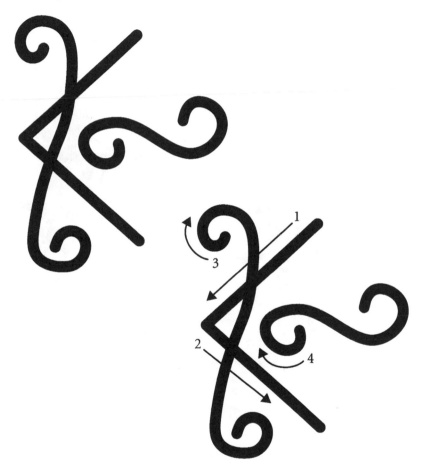

Figure 26: Shanti

Om

Om is not a channeled symbol, but an ancient Sanskrit symbol that has been adopted by the Karuna traditions. Om is the sound of creation, more accurately spelled "AUM," with the three letters symbolizing the creative, stabilizing and destructive principles of the universe. In Hinduism, the forces are personified as Brahma, Vishnu, and Shiva, but the concept can be found in many other cultures. Om symbolizes all of creation, a symbol of oneness and unity. The detached dot symbolizes the one true essence, detached from its creation, and the symbol can be used to bring detachment. It is the Master symbol of the Karuna traditions, and is used in sessions to bring a sense of oneness, open the crown chakra when blocked, and cleanse the aura.

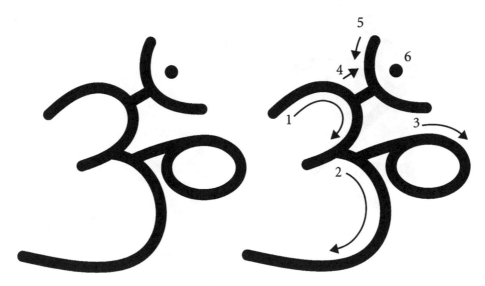

Figure 27: Om

Mer Ka Fa Ka Lish Ma

Mer Ka Fa Ka Lish Ma is a symbol of the Shamballa tradition, manifesting the power of the divine Mother. I love this symbol because it represents so many powerful magickal symbols. Within it is the ankh, the Egyptian symbol of life, representing the unity of the god Osiris and goddess Isis, as well as the Greek caduceus, representing the chakras and, in a modern sense, the DNA symbol and the Christian peace symbol. Mer Ka Fa Ka Lish Ma is used to align one to the perfect pattern of health, healing DNA, reconnecting with the divine Goddess, aligning the chakras, and healing the Earth.

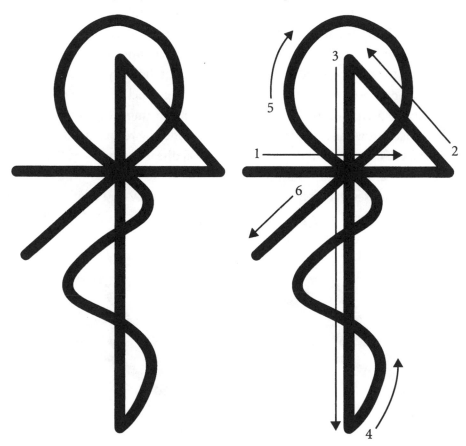

Figure 28: Mer Ka Fa Ka Lish Ma

Motor Zanon

Motor Zanon is found under a variety of names and is believed to be of Tibetan or Sanskrit origin. Kathleen Milner states that at least one Tibetan monk uses the symbol for exorcisms. Although it resembles the Tibetan Master symbol, it is very different in form and function. In some traditions of Reiki, it is called the Anti-Viral symbol. Energetically, it acts like a viral magnet. Empower it with Cho Ku Rei by drawing Cho Ku Rei and chanting its name three times, then draw this symbol, chanting Motor three times, and then draw and chant Cho Ku Rei again. Imagine pushing the symbol into the recipient's body. The "corkscrew" spins, attracting viral particles, filling the funnel shape. Use your intuition to know when to take it out, and when ready, chant Cho Ku Rei three times, followed by Zanon three times, and then Cho Ku Rei three times again. This reverses the action, drawing the symbol, filled with viral energy, out of the body. "Destroy" the symbol either with symbols used to break apart unwanted energy, such as Cho Ku Rei/Sei He Ki combinations, or perhaps Halu, or simply visualize it burning away in a white or violet flame. You must remove and heal this energy. Once done, the recipient will notice a great decline in the viral disease. Although it can heal viral disease completely, the underlying issues must be healed as well. To be honest, I didn't believe this at all when I learned it, but I've used it with several clients, in particular one with HIV and another with herpes, and the symbol has been very powerful in managing, if not curing, their illnesses. I've also used it on the flu with almost immediate effects.

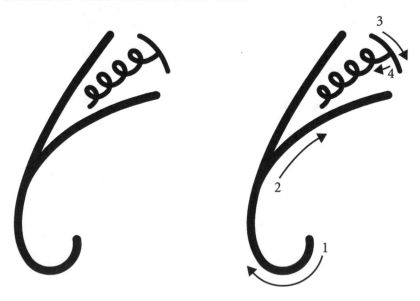

Figure 29: Motor Zanon

Hosanna

Hosanna is drawn in two different ways. The first version sends out a clearing energy. The second version focuses on a specific issue the client wants to heal. A clearing technique combines Hosanna with an invocation of St. Michael, the Angels of the Violet Flame, and St. Germain, but you can simply use it with clear intent. This symbol is credited to Eileen Gurhy of New York, NY.

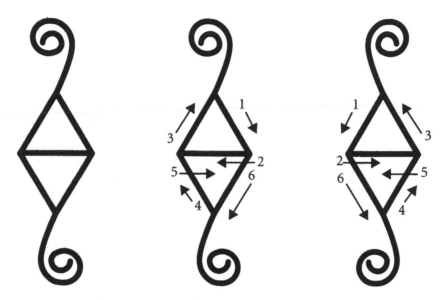

Figure 30: Hosanna Clearing and Hosanna Healing

Johre®

The Johre® symbol is a variation of the Japanese calligraphy symbol of the Johre® Foundation. Literally, it is said to mean "white light." It puts white light wherever it is used, helps the recipient release what doesn't serve, opens the chakras, and connects to spirit guides and ascended masters.

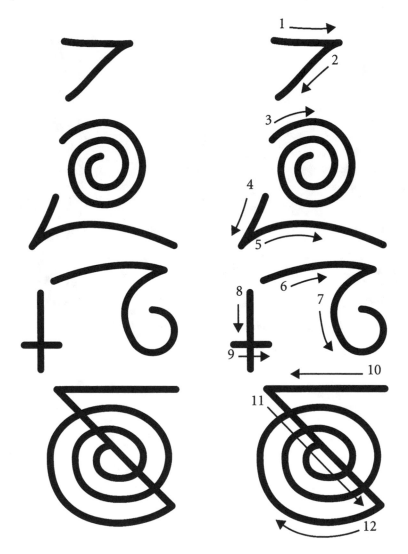

Figure 31: Johre®

Om Benza Satto Hung

This mantra and symbol is used for purification. It brings up harmful energies to be transmuted, and can be used in both meditation and healing sessions. Continue repeating the mantra and visualizing the symbol. In the Tera Mai™ traditions, it is used to remove unwanted energies and what are considered to be "humanly contrived initiations" from other traditions.

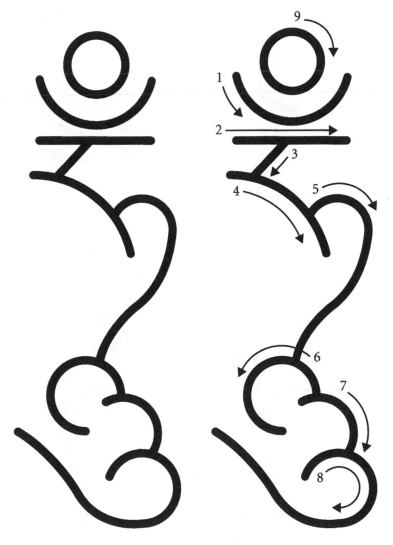

Figure 32: Om Benza Satto Hung

Palm Master Symbol

The Palm Master symbol, also known as the Palm Di Ko Mio, is seen on the palms of many statues in the East, signifying the healing power of those palms. Now it is used as a symbol in the Shamballa tradition, both in the hands and for the entire chakra system. It is said to symbolize the chakra system: point 1 is the crown, 2 connects to the third eye, 3 is the throat, 4 moves through other chakras to the Earth, and 5 connects to the higher chakras beyond the open crown.

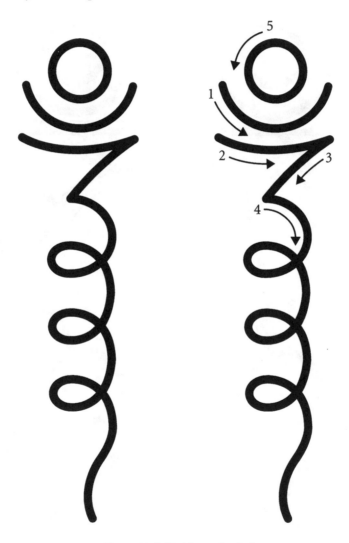

Figure 33: Palm Master Symbol

Dai Zon

Dai Zon (often pronounced "di-don") means "from my heart to your heart." I know that several Reiki Masters in New England use it, but haven't seen it much elsewhere. Some call it by this name, while others simply use it as the "opening spiral." They use it to start a session, spiraling out from the heart through the chakras. Dia Zon is credited to Lyn Roberts-Herrick, a teacher of Shamanic Reiki.

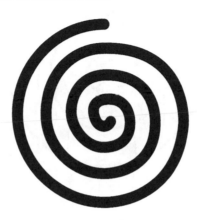

Figure 34: Dai Zon

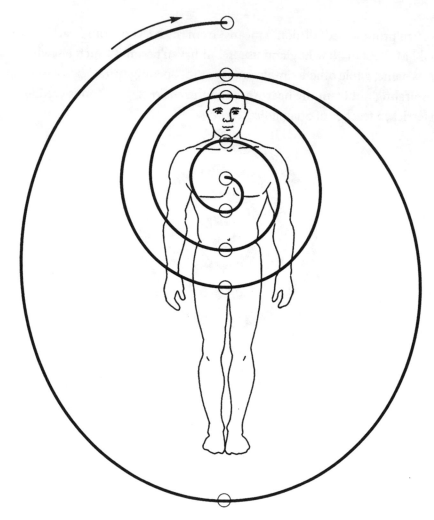

Figure 35: Drawing Dai Zon: Heart, Solar Plexus, Throat, Belly, Brow, Root, Crown, Earth Star, Soul Star

Cho Ku Ret

Cho Ku Ret is the Power symbol of the Seichim traditions, transforming the spiraling energy of Cho Ku Rei with the infinity loop. Cho Ku Ret is not only used for healing people, but also healing noncellular beings, such as crystals, and for healing machines, cars, and computers. The spiritual lesson behind Cho Ku Ret is that everything is alive and filled with the same energy as we are.

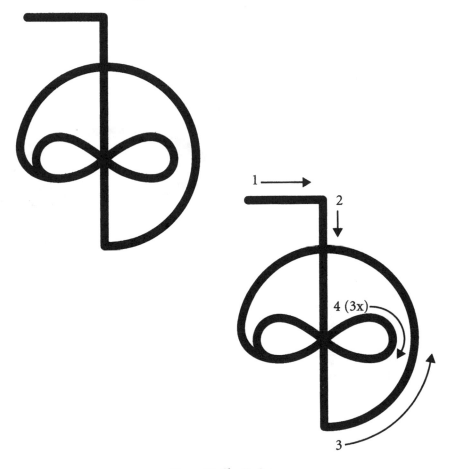

Figure 36: Cho Ku Ret

Angel Wings

Another Seichim symbol, Angel Wings is used to help you realize your potential, your own angelic divinity, and bring that out into the world. Angel Wings connects the user to the realm of angels, guides, guardians, and healers. It also brings the protection of the angels.

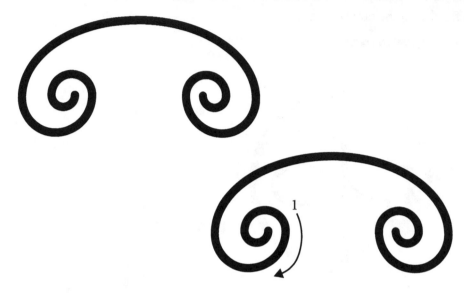

Figure 37: Angel Wings

Male Female

Our third Seichim symbol balances male and female energies, regardless of our physical gender. It soothes relations with the opposite sex, helping us to see a partner's point of view, and helps those struggling with the limited gender identities of our society.

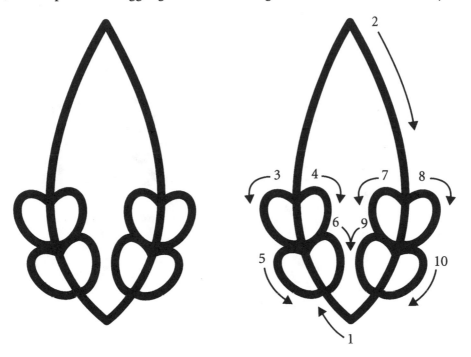

Figure 38: Male Female

High Low God Selves

While the Male Female symbol balances our gender polarity, this Seichim symbol balances our higher self and ego self, bringing a great sense of wisdom. Another variation of this symbol is called Christ Light, and is used to bring the highest ideals of love and spirit to the user, and then the user can to act upon them.

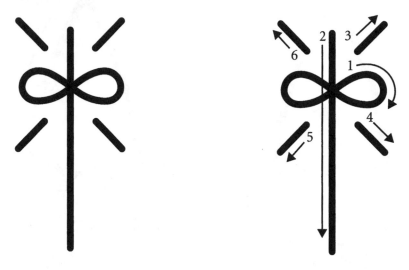

Figure 39: High Low God Selves

Eeeeftchay

Eeeeftchay is the Seichim symbol of "endless inner sight," bringing clarity to any issue. Used on any chakra, it brings inner sight and clarity to issues of that chakra. Eeeeftchay also opens our natural psychic abilities when used on the third eye.

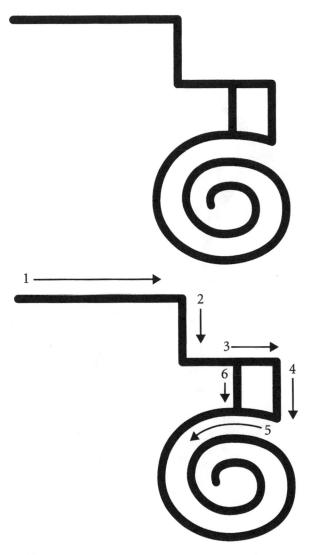

Figure 40: Eeeeftchay

Len So My

Len So My is the power of pure love, and is used when an individual needs to feel pure, unconditional love when feeling lost, neglected, or unwanted.

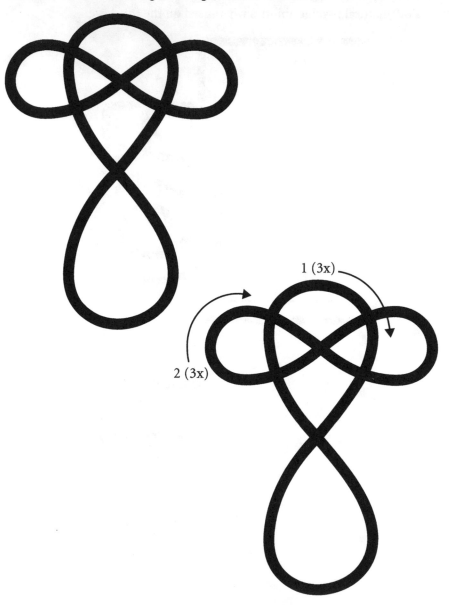

Figure 41: Len So My

Lon Say

Not much information is available regarding Lon Say. The only formal meanings I've encountered say "infection negativity." These words can be interpreted in two ways. I prefer to think of it as cleansing an infection, not infecting one with negative energy. The symbol can be used when "negative" or unwanted energies take root, to clear out this imbalanced infection. The symbol can also be used for any type of physical infection, which ultimately is the process of unwanted energies taking root. When guided, I've used Lon Say down the entire body, starting at the crown. It tends to balance the different sides of the body, including the arms and legs, but focuses on the center spiral in the chest area. It also seems to soothe abdominal issues, gently sweeping them out with the four wave-like lines.

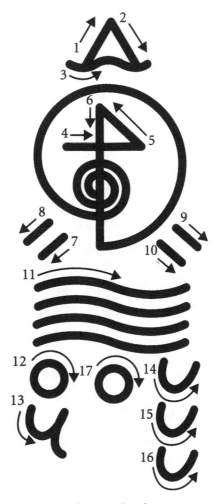

Figure 42: Lon Say

Yod

Yod is a powerful yet strange symbol. It is said to be the energy of the caretaker of the heart, and connected to the myth of the Ark of the Covenant. It is also used to connect to higher guidance and psychic ability through the heart. Kathleen Milner uses it in conjunction with her Egyptian Cartouche Initiation, to help diviners gain a stronger understanding of archetypal energies.

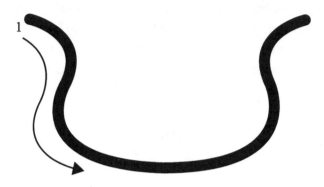

Figure 43: Yod

Chakra Symbols

The chakra symbols are symbols and mantras traditionally associated with the seven major energy centers identified in Hindu traditions. Each mantra is the "seed sound" of the chakra, discovered by the yogis and gurus upon meditation. The symbols have made their way into many Reiki traditions, to heal and balance each particular chakra. The symbols represent the basic energy of the chakra, much like the colors of each chakra. Draw them as intuitively guided, or simply visualize them. The use of color, mantra, and symbol, in any and all combinations, helps align and heal the chakras, quieting overactive chakras and energizing low-energy chakras.

OM	Crown	Inspiration/divinity
KSHAM	Brow	Intuition/vision
HAM	Throat	Expression/will
YAM	Heart	Balance/love
RAM	Solar Plexus	Wholeness/energy/self-esteem
VAM	Belly	Stability/trust
LAM	Root	Potency/grounding

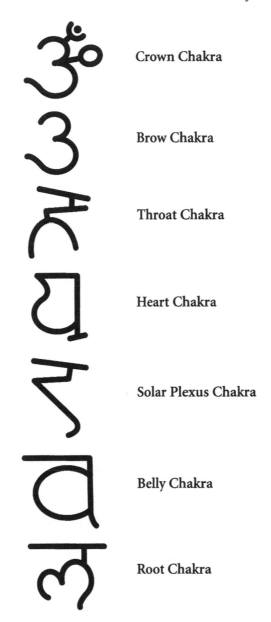

Crown Chakra

Brow Chakra

Throat Chakra

Heart Chakra

Solar Plexus Chakra

Belly Chakra

Root Chakra

Figure 44: Chakra Symbols

These symbols are traditionally viewed from the crown to the root. I was given them by a Reiki Master to use in healing, but never given specific ways to draw them.

Amsui Symbols

The Amsui symbols are used in the attunement process of Shamballa. Each is an individual symbol (note the repeating of stroke 1), although they are usually used in this pattern. The Amsui symbols signify completion and aid in the completion and integration of the attunement process. As the energies of the Earth become more spiritual, the Amsui symbols used in the Shamballa attunement process and healing sessions help the Shamballa healing energies change to match the new vibrations of the Earth and her inhabitants. Without them, the healing energies might remain static as the Earth and her people continue to evolve. Some practitioners use the Amsui symbols to signify the completion of a session. They can be used whenever anyone is going through an energetic change and needs to adapt. This channeled symbol is credited to Bas Van Woelderen.

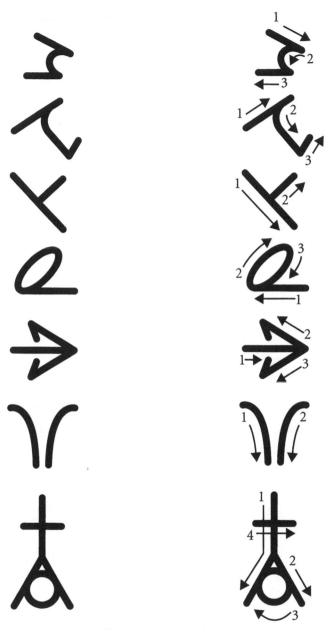

Figure 45: Amsui Symbols

Abundance

This symbol was given to me in my Shamballa Three and Four class as a symbol to manifest abundance in life, or help one heal issues of poverty consciousness and bring in prosperity consciousness. I find it interesting that this symbol is very similar to the astrological glyph for Sagittarius (♐). Sagittarius, the archer, is the sign associated with the planet Jupiter. In ceremonial magick, Jupiter is the planet of abundance, good fortune, good business, and expansion.

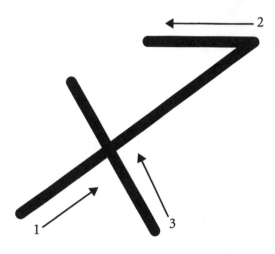

Figure 46: Abundance

Ho Ka O ili ili

This symbol was given to me in my Shamballa Three and Four class as a symbol to increase regality and respect. If we have low self-esteem or a poor self-image, or if we are not relating well to others, this symbol can help us stand up for our basic rights and gain respect. When chanted, each vowel is pronounced separately. To me, the sound of Ho Ka O ili ili is similar in dialect to Hawaiian when you first hear it.

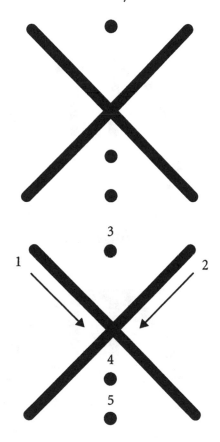

Figure 47: Ho Ka O ili ili

Anti-Cancer Symbol

This symbol is drawn into the body, or above the body and pushed into it. It heals the body of malignant growths, such as cancer, and promotes the growth of normal, healthy cells. Place Anti-Cancer wherever there is malignant cell growth. This Shamballa symbol was received by Loril Moondream, who, affiliated with the White Mountain Apache, used Native American teachings, Reiki, and visioning techniques in obtaining the symbols she has shared with me in this book. They were given to her personally in a vision, and are not traditional tribal symbols.

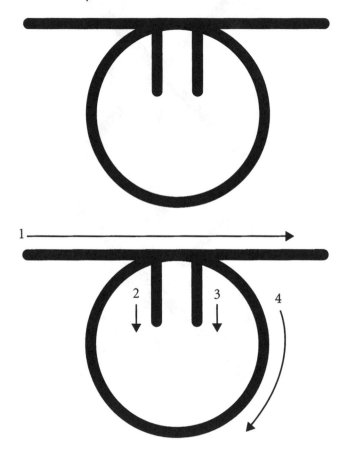

Figure 48: Anti Cancer Symbol

Heal the Healers

This symbol brings the energy of Quan Yin, the mother energy of compassion and unconditional love. It is to be used by healers on themselves and other healers, so all may learn to take time for the self. This Shamballa symbol was received by Loril Moondream.

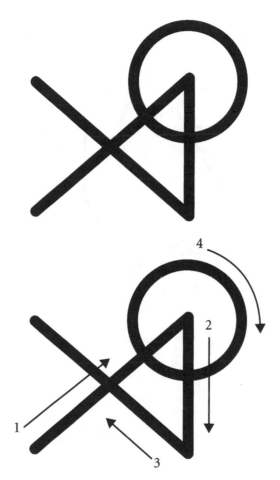

Figure 49: Heal the Healers

Twelve-Pointed Star

The Twelve-Pointed Star is used in the heart chakra during Shamballa attunements. The heart is often symbolized by a six-pointed star, so the twelve points are an amplification of this heart energy, as well as being symbolic of the twelve signs of the zodiac. In sacred geometry, the twelve-sided Platonic solid, the dodecahedron, corresponds to the element of Spirit. You can use this shape, drawn or visualized, in any chakra healing work. It is also used with crystal points in a healing mandala for both people and the Earth.

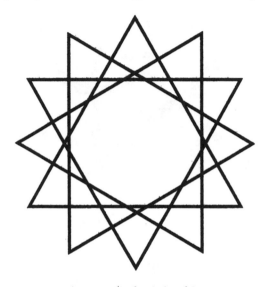

Figure 50: Twelve-Pointed Star

Flower of Life

Another symbol used in the Shamballa attunement process, the Flower of Life is said to represent the geometry of the divine. The two-dimensional Flower of Life is a series of nineteen interlocking circles from which all the sacred Platonic solids can be derived. Some versions of it continue the pattern beyond the first nineteen circles, creating a six-petaled flower in each of the nineteen circles. The founder of Shamballa, Hari Das, says that the Flower of Life is the "seed blue print for life," representing the divine plan, highest good, and perfect health. You can visualize the two- or three-dimensional Flower of Life in a session, or around the healing space.

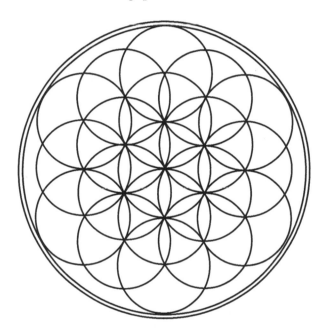

Figure 51: Flower of Life

As you can tell, some symbols are very specific, and others are very general. Many repeat themselves in function. The symbols are not absolutes, but representations of vast archetypal energies. Use them as a gateway to make your own sacred connections to these healing powers.

These are the most popular symbols I've worked with and seen others use in a variety of Reiki traditions. If you want more inspiration to connect with the divine and receive your own symbols through Reiki, look to the additional symbols in appendix 1.

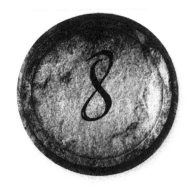

Reiki Magick

Now you know the basics of both magick and Reiki, but what is Reiki magick? For me, Reiki magick is a natural extension of these two arts. I was involved in both and viewed them as separate disciplines, but they aren't. The energies animating both of them come from the same source. The application, the techniques, and even some of the philosophies are so similar that I can't understand how there can be such a schism between the two. Most people in the Reiki community have preconceived notions about magick, and those in the magickal communities often think of Reiki as a fluffy, New Age tradition, with little substance. Both groups need to widen their view.

When I was taking my Reiki Two class, on a lunch break, we sat around the table eating. Our teacher couldn't open a jar. The lid was stuck tight. She used it as an opportunity to teach us something that isn't found in Reiki manuals. She showed us how the Power and Mental/Emotional symbols, in combination, can be used to remove all kinds of blocks, not just blocks to healing. She drew and chanted the symbols over the jar, and the lid twisted right off, like magick! From my point of view, it literally was magick—using energy, intent, and symbol to create a change in accord with your will. Was it for the highest good that the jar lid came off? You could make that argument if you wanted to, but more important to me was her intent and the method she chose to direct it—Reiki.

Now, opening a jar lid seems like a pretty silly example of spiritual magick, but magick at its heart is practical, and if you can't eat, you can't move further along your path. A lot of tribal magick was originally for eating—rain for the plants, blessings for a fruitful harvest, spells for the hunters to find the herd—so an act of magick to open a stuck jar fits right into my worldview.

That experience stuck in my mind and broadened my perspective. In my Reiki Two and Reiki Teacher level classes, we learned all sorts of ways to use Reiki that seemed very ritualistic and magickal to me, including prayer, song, affirmations, protection, blessings, and crystals. Reiki training didn't seem that different from my witchcraft training; it was simply a different method of delivery.

For a brief time, I was part of an online community that discussed the concept of using magick and Reiki together, fusing the concepts of Chaos magick to the system. They called it Chaos Reiki, which wasn't a very healing name to me, but I understood the idea. It was great to have a community of people using Reiki in different ways, exploring and sharing their experiences. Then I was introduced to several witches, like myself, who were also Reiki practitioners. They discussed how they used Reiki in their craft, candle magick, herbalism, and even cooking. I found the experience wonderful and continued my exploration, formulating my own thoughts on Reiki magick.

Witchcraft and magick were already an integral part of my life, as my spiritual path, and it was hard for me to incorporate Reiki in the same way, because I thought initially that Reiki was separate from magick. Now I know that they go together quite well, and whether intentional or not, magick and Reiki are present in everything I do.

Safeguards

The Reiki system, through the Usui lineage, has inherent "safeguards" built into it. The energy is guided by higher intelligence. The energy cannot be used to harm others because the recipient of it, or rather the recipient's higher self, is in charge of the process. Some Reiki traditions don't think of it as the higher self, but a natural body wisdom, that controls the process. Your cells and organs naturally know what to do. They even know how much Reiki to "suck" in and when to stop. The Reiki practitioner is simply the vehicle of transfer, like the straw being sucked.

Magick, on the other hand, has no safeguards. It is ruled by intent. The ultimate practice is to connect with the divine will, the higher self of the practitioner. Ceremonial magicians call this the marriage to the Holy Guardian Angel. But on the road to that union, magickal practitioners must learn to live with the consequences of all their actions, magickal or otherwise.

A part of most magickal traditions is a vow of some sort to the highest good. In Wicca, the premise is the Wiccan Rede: "An it harm none, do what ye Will." Certain ceremonial magick traditions, inspired by Aleister Crowley's *Book of the Law,* have: "Do what thou Will shall be the whole of the Law. Love is the Law. Love under Will." Each tradition may have a different way of phrasing it, but the oath is to the highest good, harming none, in unconditional love. Most magickal traditions believe that whatever you send out returns to you, creating magick. This is the premise of all spell work. The intentions and thoughts you put out return to you, creating magick.

So how can two systems, one with inherent safeguards and one without, intersect and work together harmoniously? Intention is the key. Intention rules all things. I wonder how much of the Reiki system truly has these inherent safeguards in it. Perhaps these safeties are not truly inherent, but were created through intention, and these philosophies of safety eventually became a foundation stone in the practice of Reiki. The energy is passed from teacher to practitioner with the understanding that it is a healing energy being used without any harm or ego. The ritual of initiation holds this intention and seems to be self-replicating with each transfer of energy. Perhaps the understanding is needed from both teacher and practitioner, or perhaps it only needed to be understood by Dr. Usui, and now it is replicated in each attunement process, regardless of any changes in the attunement process because the energy is the same.

I know that when I first learned witchcraft, we learned to meditate each day, and the first thing we said to ourselves, programming our consciousness, was, "At this level, everything I do is correct and for the good of all, harming none." That has become an inherent safeguard for me.

In the end, practitioners of both magick and Reiki should hold the intention of the highest good.

Attunement as Mystical Technology

The attunement process is not solely found in Reiki. An attunement is an initiation, as many esoteric traditions have energetic transfers and initiations. Modern, nontraditional

Reiki Masters have used the attunement process, the technology and ritual, to create new energies, traditions, and magickal effects.

Kathleen Milner, the founder of Tera Mai™, uses an attunement process with Egyptian archetypes, as she has been guided to use, called the Cartouche Initiation. Through this initiation, the recipient gains a greater understanding of archetypal forces. The recipient makes a leap in understanding and interpreting the archetypes of any divination or oracle system. After initiation, practitioners of Tarot, runes, ogham, and other types of divination report a greater awareness in using these systems.

Others have used the attunement process to "attune" another to the Norse runes, Celtic ogham, and other symbol systems. People have attuned others to symbols they have psychically received, and to traditional symbols, such as the cross, triangle, infinity symbol, triskallion, pentagram, pentacle, hexagram, and ankh.

Some people don't feel they need to be attuned to Reiki to do Reiki. Most say this because they don't understand the process and nature of Reiki. Others who are well versed in the history of Reiki point out that Dr. Usui didn't receive an attunement from a Reiki Master. He received a direct, spontaneous initiation from the divine. If he got that, couldn't anybody? Couldn't anyone with an open heart and mind receive such a gift from the divine? The answer is, I don't know. That's not how it happened to me and most people I know, but who am I to say that no one else has received a spontaneous attunement? In my experience, it isn't likely to happen.

Another interesting question is whether or not an attunement lasts between lifetimes. If you feel you were attuned to Reiki, in some form or tradition, in a previous lifetime, are you still attuned? Is the attunement in your body or your soul? Can you take it with you? In the Hindu traditions, some say only a true enlightened master-teacher can awaken your kundalini, the energy of awareness. Kundalini is described as a sleeping serpent at the root, waiting to be awakened through the chakras to bring greater awareness, though there is a lot of fear around kundalini awakenings in some literature. If a master has awakened your kundalini in any lifetime, it can be reawakened without the master in any lifetime afterward. I have a friend who believes that Reiki works the same way. Perhaps Reiki attunements awakens kundalini energy as well.

In my experience, people who claim to still be attuned to Reiki from a previous lifetime, but who have not experienced a physical attunement in this lifetime, have some difficulties. Perhaps their spiritual bodies are attuned, but some physical problems arise.

They seem to lack those inherent physical safeguards that protect them from taking on illness or draining their own physical bodies. These friends seem to get sick, feeling nauseous and getting headaches, so I don't suggest working from this paradigm. A simple Reiki attunement removes any inherent dangers in this process.

Distance Attunements

Through our discussion in chapter 4 of the concepts of the Distance symbol, Hon Sha Ze Sho Nen, you know that it is possible to send Reiki energy and Reiki symbols over a distance. This theory has been expanded to include attunements. Such thoughts are controversial in the Reiki community. Some feel a teacher is needed in person to transfer the energy and teachings. Others feel it is a way to keep Reiki a business and prevent it from being shared freely. In the end, I think it depends on how the process is run by the teacher. I know of quite a few online Reiki courses, with distance attunements, that are as comprehensive as any in-person course I've seen, and some are even better than some slapdash in-person trainings. As in everything, your experience will vary depending on with whom you work.

The most common kind of distance attunements are healing attunements. Like traditional healing attunements, they can be done as part of a whole distant treatment, or alone. The Tibetan Reiki tradition uses distance healing attunements, but does not generally encourage distance practitioner attunements. But if it is possible to do a distance healing attunement, then it is equally possible for a practitioner attunement to be passed via distance.

To do any type of a distance attunement, simply use the Distance symbol to open a "gateway" as you would in a distant treatment and send the symbols once you have permission. The one passing the attunement can ask the recipient to make a space and time to meditate and receive the energy. The practitioner can send symbols through the Distance symbol gateway, or can use a surrogate, like a pillow, teddy bear, or the knee, as in the distance techniques. Through this technique, it is possible to do a healing attunement on yourself. I have found this to be very powerful, and I highly suggest it! I personally am not in favor of distance practitioner attunements for my own practice, since I prefer in-person teaching to online and phone teaching, but if it is something you are drawn to, I encourage you to follow your intuition and guidance.

Reiki Ritual

One of the most effective magickal techniques is ritual. Some people don't like the word ritual, feeling it's too occult sounding, and prefer the word ceremony. I learned that a ceremony is ritual with two or more people, so I often use the words synonymously. A ritual or ceremony is basically a symbolic action to direct energy. All religious rites, magickal or otherwise, have a basis in ritual, from the Native American rain dances to the Catholic Mass. All are symbolic acts that create change, whether the change is in the external or internal world.

The first formal magickal ritual I learned is called the Magick Circle, or the Witch's Circle. The purpose of the circle is to create a sacred space for meditation, healing, and spell work. During the circle ritual, the four directions are faced, one by one, inviting the powers of the directions as embodied by the elements Earth, Fire, Air, and Water to guard and guide those in the sacred space. Many find aspects of this ceremony very similar to the rituals of Native North and South Americans who honor the four directions and elements in their own rituals. Most traditions that honor the Earth in some way honor the four directions as well as the Moon, Sun, and stars.

When I took Reiki Two, I learned a ritual different from the Magick Circle, but it has a very similar purpose and technique. The double Cho Ku Rei is drawn, with the "flags" pointing in, creating a doorway-like image, in the four directions. The intention is for them to seal the space, letting only the most healing and loving energies into or out of the space. The double Cho Ku Rei is also drawn on the ceiling above and the floor below. With those six directions, the space is sealed. Then Cho Ku Rei and Sei He Ki are drawn in the center, to clear the space of all remaining unwanted, harmful, or dense energies. Any other additional symbols known, particularly Hon Sha Ze Sho Nen and, if at the Master level, the Master symbols, are drawn. This creates a sealed, clear, sacred space to do healing sessions or classes. You can also use it to clear out the "bad vibes" of any place that needs healing or cleansing. I use it as a part of my "psychic" house cleaning of my home, office, and car, particularly if any emotionally charged events, arguments, or releases have occurred, so the energy of such releases does not linger and taint future events.

With both rituals you have the option of using cleansing incense prior to the creation of sacred space, such as sage, frankincense/myrrh, lavender, or copal. I found so many similarities between the two rituals. The magick circle is more intense and intricate and requires not only an opening ritual, but also, when it is done, a proper closing and releasing ritual to close all the elemental gateways and release the sacred space. The Reiki sealing/cleansing does not require a closing. Its effects simply fade after a session.

Combining the best of both rituals, I've used the Reiki Circle, described in the next section, to create a sacred space, particularly in situations where those involved would not be comfortable with traditional ceremonial magick. It creates a safe space for healing, counseling, meditation, prayer, and magick.

For such rituals, it is often customary to have an altar, a magickal workspace, but it is not a requirement. A simple altar can consist of a table with items symbolic of the four elements. You could have a stone or crystal for Earth in the North; a red candle for Fire in the East; incense or sage for Air in the South; and a bowl, chalice, or seashell for Water in the West. I usually place a white candle in the center for Spirit. Use the symbols and arrangement you desire.

Reiki Circle

Orient yourself in your space and, if possible, stand facing the North. Point your hand at the North and allow the Reiki energy to flow out to the perimeter of the room or wherever you want the boundary of the sacred space to be. (It can be through the walls or even beyond them.) Visualize the energy beaming from your hand, and turn clockwise, creating a ring of energy around the space. Do this three times in total, with the intention of creating a sacred space.

Face the North. Draw the double Cho Ku Rei doorway and empower the symbols by chanting their name three times. Then say:

"To the North, I invite the healers of the Earth and the Body to be present. Hail and welcome."

Face the East. Draw the double Cho Ku Rei doorway and empower the symbols by chanting their name three times. Then say:

"To the East, I invite the healers of Fire and the Soul to be present. Hail and welcome."

Face the South. Draw the double Cho Ku Rei doorway and empower the symbols by chanting their name three times. Then say:

> *"To the South, I invite the healers of Air and the Mind to be present. Hail and welcome."*

Face the West. Draw the double Cho Ku Rei doorway and empower the symbols by chanting their name three times. Then say:

> *"To the West, I invite the healers of Water and the Heart to be present. Hail and welcome."*

Now you have created a sacred space, and can do any of the techniques discussed in this chapter and subsequent chapters. Everything magickal is enhanced when in a sacred space. Take care not to leave the bounds of the sacred space until you release it.

When done, the space must be released by starting in the North and reversing your actions, going counterclockwise. You don't have to draw any Reiki symbols to release, but you can if you desire. Follow the same process, but reverse it.

> *"To the North, I thank and release the healers of the Earth and Body. Hail and farewell.*
>
> *To the West, I thank and release the healers of Water and the Heart. Hail and farewell.*
>
> *To the South, I thank and release the healers of Air and the Mind. Hail and farewell.*
>
> *To the East, I thank and release the healers of Fire and the Soul. Hail and farewell."*

Face the North again, raising your hands, and move counterclockwise once, imagining the ring of light expanding out infinitely.

Reiki Consecration

Practitioners of magickal traditions believe in the power of imbuing objects with energy and intention. Such actions are called consecrating, charging, blessing, or hallowing. Simply through intention, energy is placed in an object to enhance its use. The wonderful thing about such objects is that they can be given to those not involved in Reiki or magick and still carry their effective power. This consecration is the source of power for the magickal charms found throughout the ages and in many lands. You can consecrate jewelry such as rings and necklaces, along with crystals and stones. Someone with a prolongued illness can wear a ring charged for healing. I have "Reiki-ed" the stones in my garden for healing and protection. I also use Reiki on all my ceremonial tools, such as my wand, blade, candles, incense, and statues.

Traditionally, mystics say that things with a more solid structure, such as metal and stone, "take" a charge of intention and energy better than others, but don't let that limit you. I use Reiki to bless my food before eating it, often using Cho Ku Rei along with Mer Ka Fa Ka Lish Ma to heal any impurities in it, as well as activate any healing properties in it. I do Reiki on my herbs and other medicines. I have also Reiki-ed stuffed animals.

Consecrate an object by holding it and letting the Reiki flow into it (hands-on Reiki) and by drawing the Reiki symbols on it. Such objects are usually cleansed first, to remove any harmful energies that might conflict with your intention. You can cleanse them with a purifying incense, or again use the combination of Cho Ku Rei, Sei He Ki, Cho Ku Rei three times. (This symbol combination removes all blocks and unwanted energies. I've even used it to unclog a toilet!) Then hold the object in your hands and feel the Reiki flow into it. Use the symbols that correspond with your intention, if you have a particular intention. You can simply put the basic Reiki Two and/or Reiki Master symbols in the object, and ask that the Reiki flow as needed, for the highest good, in accord with the user's need.

Reiki Moon Magick

Once while teaching a Reiki class, I had a student who wanted nothing to do with magick or witchcraft. She enjoyed my other classes, but felt such things were against her religion and she was uncomfortable with it. I can understand and respect her feelings. Then she taught me Reiki Moon magick, though she didn't call it that. She said her first Reiki teacher had taught her this technique, and she didn't understand why I was so surprised. I explained to her she had been doing magick all along, just Reiki magick, and that magick can be found in many cultures and religions, including Judaism, Christianity, and Islam.

The basic technique consists of writing out a "wish list" of material objects you desire or events you wish to occur, with the intention that they occur only for the highest good. These statements should be written in a positive manner, not from a place of want or lack. They should read as if they had already happened, or were in the process of happening. Such a list could look like this:

I have a new job that fulfills all my financial and personal needs.

I have a perfectly healthy heart and circulatory system.

I have a new car stereo.

I am happy in my home life.

The list can be as long or as short as you would like. At first it seems like a list of simple affirmations found in many traditions, from the mystical to the self-help world, but here is the most interesting magickal part. This person suggested it be timed with the Moon phase, a long-time magickal tradition. She suggested starting the list when the Moon begins to wax, or grow in light from the new Moon to the first quarter. When the Moon is increasing in light, it is the time to do magick with the intention to create, grow, or manifest. When the Moon is waning, or decreasing in light, it is the time to banish, remove, or protect.

Start the list as the light of the Moon starts to grow. Every day, hold the list between your hands and do hands-on Reiki on the list, filling the paper with energy as you chant "Cho Ku Rei" over and over again. Do this for anywhere from a few minutes to fifteen minutes a day. You can visualize or draw the symbol over the list. You don't necessarily have to read the list every day. In fact, its best if you don't, to simply let the energy build without attachment.

When the Moon is full, do Reiki on your list one last time. When you are done, burn or bury the list and let your intention manifest in your life.

The process can be reversed to create a list of things you would like to banish. Here is an example:

I banish my fear of flying.

I banish any illness in my digestive system.

I banish all pain in my knee.

I banish the legal dispute between me and my former spouse.

Begin the list after the full Moon and build to a peak at the new Moon, burning or burying the list at that time.

Although I like the list concept and believe that the universal life force is ever abundant, sometimes I need to focus on just one intention to manifest in my life. In witchcraft, I use this format for spell work when the Moon is waxing:

"I, (State your personal or spiritual name), ask in the name of the Goddess and God to be granted (State your intention). I thank the Goddess and God for all favors and ask that this be correct, for the highest good, harming none. So mote it be."

If the Moon is waning, rephrase the first sentence to read: *"I ask in the name of the Goddess and God to remove (State your intention)."* You can use any name for the divine if you are not comfortable with "the Goddess and God." The phrase "So mote it be" simply means "So be it" or "It is so." Witches use it like a final affirmation, to say that this is so, it has already happened, and I thank you for it. Using it is like making a positive affirmation. Here is an example of a traditional waxing Moon spell:

"I, Christopher, ask in the name of the Goddess and God to be granted a new garden space acceptable to me, and the time to work and play in it. I thank the Goddess and God for all favors, and ask that this be correct, for the highest good, harming none. So mote it be."

Use either the list or the specific intention format, and feel free to adapt them to suit your own personal magickal style.

The Reiki Box

The Reiki box is another technique I learned that struck me as being very similar to traditional magick. In witchcraft, there is a folk magick technique called a spell box, or more modernly a manifestation bowl. A box or bowl is used as a vessel, and is cleansed and blessed in ritual, with the intention of manifesting any wish that is placed in it. Names of people in need of healing and guidance are placed in it, as well as spells and intentions. Crystals (see chapter 11) and dried herbs or roots (see chapter 12) that match the intentions of the work can also be added. Such spell boxes should be started at the new Moon. The box is placed on the altar or other place used to meditate, and intention and energy are placed into the box, "recharging" it each day. If a new need arises, another "wish" paper is added to the spell box. The entire process lasts for either half of a Moon cycle, until the full Moon, or for an entire Moon cycle, from new Moon to new Moon. Then the contents of the box are burned or buried, and the process is begun again.

I discovered Reiki practitioners who do "Reiki boxes." They have beautifully decorated boxes, and in them they place their manifestations list and prayer list of people or places in need of Reiki healing. They place the box between their hands and Reiki it for one minute or up to a full session every day, as a part of their daily spiritual practice.

Exercise: Create a Reiki Box

Create and use a Reiki box, as just described. Cleanse it and consecrate it in your own ritual of sacred space, or use the Reiki Circle ritual described earlier in the chapter. Make this technique a part of your spiritual practice.

Reiki Candle Magick

Legend has it that Dr. Usui used to burn magickal healing candles during his Reiki healing sessions. That is a bit of lore passed among certain Reiki Masters, but I don't know if it is true. If he did, though, I think it's a wonderful idea. I had been using candle magick in my life for years before I learned Reiki. Burning wax has a magickal quality to it, and is simple to use. I know many people who have had wonderful experiences with candle magick, and I love to teach it. Then I met witches who specifically got their Reiki attunements not to focus on Reiki healing, but to enhance their candle magick and their ability to consecrate magickal items, herbs, and crystals. I had never thought about learning Reiki specifically for that purpose, but it is an excellent idea and helped inspire this book.

Candle magick is so powerful because inherent in the technique are the four elements. The wax is symbolic of the element Earth. The dripping, melted wax, and the moisture collected on it, is the Water element. The flame is obviously the Fire element, and the oxygen that feeds the flame is the Air element. The color of the candle influences the magick as well. Choose a color that you intuitively feel suits your intention. (See appendix 3 for more color information.) You have a powerful, balanced, sacred tool in the candle, and its effects are powerful alone or as part of a larger ritual.

Basic candle magick is like consecrating the candle. I learned to put magickal symbols on the candle by using a pin or knife, etching them into the wax. You can gently heat the pin or blade to make a better etching. Although some Reiki traditions would consider this sacrilegious, I now also carve Reiki symbols into the wax.

Witches and magicians infuse the candle either with their personal energy, or they draw upon the energy of the environment. If you are Reiki-attuned, you can infuse the candle with the universal life force. It's like filling a glass with water. The candle is like an empty glass, and through your carvings and simply by holding it in your hands and letting the Reiki flow, you are filling it with magickal power. Just like Reiki will flow as needed, and when it is done it stops, the candle will fill up with Reiki energy, and when it is "full" the flow stops. Then light the candle to send out your magickal intention. The flame acts like a magickal beacon, a transmitter to amplify the energy you invested into the candle and manifest your intention.

Mystical lore will tell you that if you blow out a candle, something awful will happen. You will offend the elementals of Air and Fire, and they will curse you. That's not true, but it will create an imbalance of the elements of the candle magick, since when you blow on it, you add Air energy. The spell will often not work out or will manifest in a way that is not exactly what you desired, seeming like a curse. So, if possible, let your candle burn all the way until it is done. If that is not practical, since you don't want to leave candles burning while you sleep or go to work, snuff the candle out without blowing or wetting it and then relight it when it is practical to do so.

Candle Healing Spell

You can use candle magick and any Reiki symbols for healing, but I like to draw Hon Sha Ze Sho Nen at the top of the candle, down the side. Then write the person's name vertically down the candle, and finish the line with Cho Ku Rei and Sei He Ki if there is room at the bottom. I usually use a green candle for basic healing, red for intense critical healing, and blue for mental and emotional healing.

Manifestation

Use candle magick with Moon magick whenever you want to manifest something in your life. I carve the candle with Cho Ku Rei, Hon Sha Ze Sho Nen, Kriya, and Abundance, with either a green or blue candle for prosperity, or a black candle to draw the energy to me, since black is the color that absorbs and attracts energy.

Past-Life Regression

When doing past-life-regression meditations and healing, I carve Zonar, Halu, and Harth down a purple or yellow candle, do Reiki on it, and burn it during such sessions.

Love

For love magick, either for self-love, divine love, or manifesting a romantic relationship, use Harth, Len So My, YAM (heart chakra symbol), and Yod down a pink or green candle.

Earth Healing

I often light a candle for healing the Earth and the people on it. My intention is not only for environmental issues, but for social and political issues, particularly in times of military conflicts. I use combinations of Mara, Iava, Mer Ka Fa Ka Lish Ma, and Johre® on a white candle.

Study

When studying for a big test of any kind, carve Gnosa, Sei He Ki, Gnosa on a blue, orange, or yellow candle to enhance understanding and memory.

Meditation

To aid meditation practices, burn a white, lavender, or purple candle with Om, Shanti, Shanti carved on it. "Om Shanti Shanti" is a traditional mantra.

Protection/Cleansing

To clear and seal a space, try using various combinations of Cho Ku Rei—Sei He Ki—Cho Ku Rei, Motor Zanon, Johre®, Len So My, and Om Benza Satto Hung with white or violet candles. You could also try Lon Say, but personally I can't draw it very well on a candle with a pin, so I don't use it much in candle magick.

Psychic Readings

When doing psychic readings such as Tarot or runes, try burning a purple or blue candle with the symbols Eeeeftchay, KSHAM (third eye chakra symbol), and Zonar on it.

Balance

If you desire balance between your inner polarities, do candle magick with the symbols Sei He Ki, Male Female, and High Low God Selves carved down the side. You must determine what color will be most balancing for you. Sometimes you can get candles in metaphysical shops that are two colors, half and half. They would be ideal for this type of spell.

Chakra Balance

To balance the chakras, for yourself or another, particularly during a healing session, place the chakra symbols from the crown at the top of the candle, down to the root at the base. Or draw the Palm Master symbol down the side. If you can acquire a rainbow candle, that would be great, but if in doubt, try a white candle.

Spiritual Guidance

To connect with higher spiritual guidance, angels, masters, and spirit guides, use the following symbols on a blue, purple, lavender, or white candle: Harth, Johre®, Angel Wings, and High Low God Selves.

Use these guides to inspire your own personal candle magick color and symbol combinations. Reiki is the universal life force, so as long as you have the intention of the highest good and harming none, feel free to experiment and play.

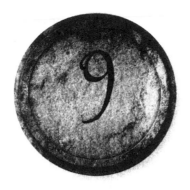

Reiki Spirit Guides

In Reiki Two, I was introduced to the concept of Reiki spirit guides. Those who use Reiki spirit guides believe that there is a group of spiritual beings who were once human, who now reside in nonphysical realms, but can interact with, and to a certain extent influence, the physical world. They are said to be Reiki practitioners from the past ages, not simply Usui Reiki practitioners who have crossed, but those from the ancient origins of Reiki. Once attuned to Reiki, you are part of the vast network, and when you are attuned, the universal life force "assigns" to you a Reiki guide to help you with your Reiki healing experiences.

Strangely enough, the concept of Reiki guides is not universal. In fact, it seems to be a New Age "add-on" found only in the Reiki traditions of the 1980s and beyond. Traditional Usui Reiki does nothing with Reiki guides, but that doesn't prevent the experience from being a reality. Much of the Usui material does not focus on the esoteric realm. I know when I took Reiki One from more conventional Usui teachers that in some ways it was more like a medical class than a mystical one. The medical approach is fine, but doesn't invalidate the experience of guides.

Psychically sensitive people involved in Reiki probably started to experience the presence of other spirits during their use of Reiki and, upon further sensing or direct communication, learned how the spirits were involved in the Reiki process. In this paradigm, they were always present in Reiki, but were never directly called upon by the more conventional practitioners. Evocation of Reiki "spirits" is not needed for Reiki itself. Reiki is simple, and I'm sure purists feel this complicates Reiki with unnecessary information and belief systems. And they are right. You don't need this material simply to do Reiki, but many people experience the phenomenon of guides after Reiki One or Two. Perhaps some are susceptible to suggestion, so if a teacher says that after Reiki Two they will meet their Reiki guide, then they have a vision or dream. I teach a meditation in Reiki Two, like my teacher before me, to help connect to the Reiki guides. But others spontaneously experience the presence of guides, and come from a belief system that doesn't explain such phenomena. The results are startling and unsettling, until you have a system to explain it and give it a place.

On the practical side, I find Reiki spirit guides to be a powerful tool. As with all spirit work, some people believe that they are just talking to an aspect of their own consciousness and giving it a shape, form, voice, and personality. That could be true. Many, however, truly believe that they are spirits from the past guiding the future, like spiritual ancestor spirits. In either case, the practitioner gets a sense of guidance, of not being alone in a situation, of having a spiritual support person or, in some cases, an entire team to guide the process. Such guidance, whatever the origin, can give a new practitioner the confidence to simply continue doing Reiki and not be scared by an intense emotional release or other healing crisis.

My Experience

Although heavily involved in the New Age and magickal worlds, I began all my explorations feeling fairly skeptical. When I got involved with spirit guides, I simply considered them a psychological device, to get a different point of view from your mind. Then, as I entered into more advanced magickal training and shamanism, I became more familiar with spirit guides and their role in my life.

So I went in with an open mind to my Reiki Two spirit guide meditation. In my heart, I was kind of expecting this little Buddhist monk in an orange robe to show up in my mind's eye. As my teacher guided us through the images, somewhat similar to the meditation later in this chapter, I came across the first guide I ever met in my magickal training. I tried to get rid of her, saying, "No, not you. I need my Reiki guide." She looked at me rather funny, and said she was my healing guide, and she could help with Reiki. She knew all about it. Didn't I think she was up to the job? When such things defy my preconceptions and expectations, I truly think I've connected to something beyond me.

During my training and later teaching, I noticed the presence of spirit guides in my healing sessions with others. I didn't recognize the image and voices as my guides, and assumed they belonged to my client. I didn't discuss this with most clients at first, but a few who are particularly sensitive psychically said they felt more than one set of hands on them at all times, or they heard people talking and whispering around them. I know they must have felt such a presence, too, and the Reiki guides were not simply a mental construct. They have a psychic energy that is perceived by others as well as the practitioner.

My most remarkable experience was with a client who was going in for surgery. I was hired to do pre- and post-op Reiki for her. I did the pre-op, but her surgeon ran late and I had a class to teach that evening. I waited as long as I could, but I couldn't stay to do the post-op Reiki. Her life partner, who is deaf, was upset, so I volunteered to attune her to Reiki One, so she could do the post-op Reiki. The partner had experienced Reiki and magick, but wasn't really involved and wasn't really sure if she believed in any of it, but she was willing to try. I attuned her and taught her the basic hand positions she would need. I kept it clinical, not mystical.

Later, she reported amazing experiences. Not only did she have the traditional hot and tingly hands, but she also reported "hearing" a voice telling her when to switch positions and where to go next. The "hearing" sensation was quite strong and startling to her, even though physically she could not hear a regular human voice. I was quite surprised and pleased that her own guidance had come through so strongly. Now I give a little more "warning" about Reiki guides to new students, and even touch upon the concept in Reiki One so that first-level students who sense a presence or hear voices don't think they are crazy. I reserve the spirit guide meditation experience for my Reiki Two class.

Who Are the Guides?

In the most conservative view, the guides are the ancestors of the lineage of Reiki. Reiki practitioners often have pictures of Usui, Hayashi, and Takata in their treatment rooms, some just out of sentiment, but I know many Masters who call upon the spirits of Usui,

Hayashi, and Takata, like a divine trinity, to guide their sessions and classes, and have a distinct sense of their presence. We can look to the Reiki Masters of the modern era who have passed from this world as potential spirit guides, as well as the souls of potential ancient Reiki practitioners from Lemuria, Atlantis, and other mystical lands.

In New Age metaphysics, spirits guides are souls who are not incarnated at this time, but are between lifetimes, helping incarnated spirits in this life. Certain schools of thought suggest that spirit guides are not souls at all, but a different type of being with the specific function to guide human souls.

Another popular concept in New Age lore is the idea of ascension. Ascension material is often tied into the Reiki world, and although they are complementary in many ways, they are not the same. I've often called Shamballa Reiki a form of "Ascension Reiki" because it stems from that paradigm. The word ascension means different things to different people. In its more basic interpretation, it means that the consciousness ascends to a higher level of spirituality and love, where one achieves what other cultures would call enlightenment, nirvana, Buddhahood, Christ consciousness, sainthood, or personal mastery. At the extreme level of interpretation, when one achieves this level of consciousness, the physical body vibrates so quickly and with so much energy that it literally disappears from this plane of reality and moves to a higher dimension. In Shamballa Reiki, Shamballa refers to the collective consciousness of the ascended beings, also called ascended masters of Earth, who guide the spiritual evolution of humanity. They are called the Great White Brotherhood in some circles, as well as the Secret Chiefs or the Order of Blessed Souls. In Shamballa Reiki, you are "assigned" an ascended master or team of masters to act as your healing guides.

The most popular form of guide for those in the general public is the angel. Practitioners call upon guardian angels, archangels, and the like to aid in healing work. Angels are not considered Reiki guides, specifically, but many who are involved in Reiki are also involved in angelic lore. Although they seem to be specifically from the Jewish, Christian, and Muslim traditions, the concept of angels can be found in the mythology and texts of Sumer, Egypt, and India. We are most familiar with the angels' Hebrew names and Judeo-Christian lore. The best-known angels are the archangels of the four directions and elements. These four archangels are referred to as the Guardians of the Watchtowers and are popular in many forms of ritual and magick.

Name	Direction	Element	Function	Description
Raphael	East	Air	Healer/Physician	Call upon to diagnose and heal the true spiritual root of the illness.
Michael	South	Fire	Protector/Warrior	Call upon to use flaming sword to cut all harmful, unwanted ties to people and the past.
Gabriel	West	Water	Messenger	Call upon to hear the messages behind any illness.
Uriel	North	Earth	Guide	Call upon to heal the physical body, or to help those cross over to the next world.

I have a special affinity for Michael and call upon him often to aid people in letting go and to protect them when feeling scared by what they are confronting on the spiritual level. One client who is very psychic didn't know I called upon the angels in her session, but said to me afterward that Michael came to her during the healing session and told her to tell me that my left hand is "the hand of Michael." I had recently noticed during the weeks before that my left hand seemed hotter and more intense than my right one and wondered why. I asked internally, and the universe gave me my answer through my client.

Meeting Your Reiki Spirit Guides

I use meditation to help people find their Reiki guides. When you feel the need to connect to this aspect of guidance, use these images to help you make contact. Start by getting into a relaxed state by lighting some candles in your meditation space. Burn any incense that relaxes you. If you use any special crystals, place them before you to set the tone.

Exercise: Reiki Spirit Guide Meditation

Start by relaxing the body from head to toe, giving each part of your body permission to relax. Then allow your mind to relax and your heart to open. When doing Reiki meditations, I often chant the name of any of the powerful symbols to get me into a more meditative state. I usually use combinations of the Usui symbols, but Harth, Johre®, and

Angel Wings are also appropriate for this meditation. Chant whatever symbol name calls to you.

Then, in your mind's eye, visualize yourself on a path. My path wanders through an old forest. Take notice of all the steps you make on the path. Take notice of any plants or animals you see, and feel the call of the path almost magnetically pull you.

As you go deeper into the path, you notice a temple in the distance. This is a Reiki healing temple. As you walk toward it, you see a closed double doorway. The doors are carved with Reiki symbols, and a bright healing light emanates from behind the door, between the cracks.

You place your hand on the door, and it gently swings open with a creak. You enter and feel yourself surrounded by light and energy. The light seems to blind you in its beauty. As you reach the center of the light, your vision clears, revealing one or more figures who are your Reiki guides.

Take a close look at your Reiki guides. Speak to them and introduce yourself. Listen to their answers with your heart, and if you can't hear them, ask them to communicate in a way you can understand. They may show you pictures or give you feelings and intuitions. Take this time to ask any questions you have about Reiki, and about your own spiritual path and practice.

When you are done, thank the Reiki guides. Ask them for a symbol, words, or another method to contact them when you need them during a session or meditations. Exit the temple and follow the path back to your conscious body awareness. Bring yourself to center within the body, and ground yourself as needed to bring your attention to the physical world.

You can return to this temple at any time to work with your guides directly, to heal, strengthen your Reiki connection, or face your shadow self. Develop your relationship with your Reiki guides, and call upon them when you need their support.

Reiki and Channeling

Reiki has not only become inexorably linked to spirit guides, but also to the phenomenon of channeling, since many people involved in channeling are also involved in Reiki. Channeling is the psychic practice of letting a spiritual entity speak through a person. Such people are referred to as channels, but in the past they were often called mediums. Now, people usually use the word medium to refer to a channel who talks exclusively to the dead.

I think channeling has become so common in the Reiki world because practitioners are said to "channel" the universal life force, but honestly, there are few similarities between the two systems. A Reiki practitioner need not be a channel, and a channel need not have anything to do with Reiki. They can complement each other, but are not part and parcel of each other. Many of the new slants on Reiki, new symbols and secret histories, come from channeled sources, which are wonderful and fascinating, but often contradictory.

Two types of channeling exist. One is called full-body channeling, where the channel's consciousness either exits the body or is suppressed, so the entity has full control over the channel's body functions, including speech. The second is conscious channeling, where the channel repeats back the message the spirit communicates, word for word, but still remains in control of the body. Conscious channels might feel like they are in a dreamlike state, but they are still present and aware in the body.

Pros and cons exist for both types of channeling. Proponents of full-body channeling say it's the only time when the channel's own ego is not present, so the message is pure. They believe that conscious channels cloud the message with their own mind and bias. Proponents of conscious channeling say the entity doesn't have a physical body for a reason and has too much energy for a physical vessel. They believe that full-body channeling burns out the chakra system of the host. They also believe that the ego is tied to the body consciousness and will be present regardless, but that if one is more conscious of it, one can filter out the ego bias and relay a truer message.

Both types of channeling work. Both kinds of channelers have given me useful information. I think the system used depends on the style of the channeler. I think conscious channeling is an extension of developing a relationship with your spirit guides and Reiki guides. I encourage you to deepen your relationship with your Reiki guides and ask for more direct information to be given to you, if you desire to explore this method of contact.

Reiki and Ghosts

Reiki can give the practitioner a greater awareness of the spirit world, but it can also be used to heal those trapped between worlds without physical bodies to touch. More and more I hear about people using Reiki for exorcisms, house protection, cleansing, and banishing unwanted spirits. To me, this is a natural extension of the healing power of Reiki.

Most cultures have a concept of ghosts, or unsettled spirits, the souls of the living who resist crossing to the next existence when the physical body dies. Sometimes these souls are obsessed with something, and are trying to finish it but can't without a body. Other times a trauma, usually an act of violence, binds them to a place. Others simply do not acknowledge that they have died. While most ghosts are created by the imagination of the viewer, and some are spiritual "echoes" reverberating in the astral plane, sometimes ghosts truly do exist.

People who suspect the presence of a ghost ask if it's a "good" ghost or a "bad" ghost. If it's good, they want to keep it. Such spirits are not pets, or even guides. Even if the ghost is not malevolent, it doesn't really belong between worlds. It is stuck and most often needs help to continue on to the next world or return to its source.

Exercise: Banishing Ritual

Banishings are rituals used to remove unwanted spirits from a location. Exorcisms are banishings to remove unwanted spirits from an individual who feels occupied by such spirits. The best way to do such rituals is to have a strong connection with your own spirit guides, who will give you the tools to help a spirit leave and cross over. Here is a simple banishing ritual, using the Reiki symbols, that you can adapt with your own guidance.

- First, meditate on the situation with your guides, asking them their opinion and permission to do this work. If the haunting serves a higher purpose, you might be told not to remove such spirits.

- Before you enter the space, say a prayer to the highest powers to protect and guide you. Call upon your Reiki guides. I would also call upon Archangel Michael for his aid.

- For each room that needs cleansing and banishing, start by placing Cho Ku Rei in the each of the four walls, and then above, below, and in the center of the room. Then draw and chant Cho Ku Rei, Sei He Ki, and Hon Sha Ze Sho Nen in the center to fill it with healing light.

- Draw Johre® in the room, to invoke a pillar of white light to guide the spirit on to its next world.

- Say a prayer, asking the spirit to return to the light, and then draw and chant Zonar, Halu, Harth, and Motor Zanon all together, until you feel the space is clear.

- Move on to the next room. When done with the entire space, thank the highest divinity, your Reiki guides, and Archangel Michael for joining you.

For more about developing a relationship with spirit guides, angels, and spirit animals, see my book *Spirit Allies: Meet Your Team from the Other Side.*

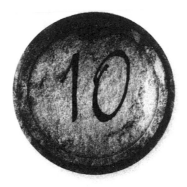

Reiki and Psychic Awakening

The magickal moment of initiation into the art of Reiki, like many spiritual initiations, often comes with an unexpected gift—an awareness of things unseen, reminiscent of the dazzling point of energetic awareness that Dr. Usui received. Those already in possession of this gift are also often drawn to study Reiki. The world at large calls this gift psychic ability, but straddles it with many misconceptions. People think when a person is psychic that this person is nearly omniscient, a mind reader capable of knowing everything about everyone. That simply isn't true. The word psychic relates to the word psyche, a concept of the soul. So a person who is psychic simply communicates with his or her own soul.

Psychic communication comes in many forms, because we all receive information differently. Some people are audio-oriented, hearing things. This gift is called clairaudience. Other people are visually oriented, and those with visual psychic skills are called clairvoyant. Others input information by simply knowing, without a real sense of words or visions. They are called clairsentient. People can have endless variations of these gifts. In fact, we all have these gifts, but have simply forgotten how to use them.

Who Is Psychic?

Before getting involved in Reiki, I taught classes on psychic development and meditation. They were a part of training people in magick and witchcraft. I think of psychic ability as a form of magick. While most people think of magick in terms of spells and charms, psychic ability is a form of information magick, and information magick is as important as any spell. Such work can help us determine if a spell should even be used in the first place. And psychic ability is a great gift to understand how everyone and everything is connected. I use psychic development to help people understand that a magickal reality is more real than they thought.

I've taught many people who absolutely insisted they were not and never would be psychic, and with practice and some fun, they had wonderful experiences. I was one of those people. I went to my teacher absolutely believing I could do nothing psychic. I felt psychic people were special people, with gifts and abilities that would be apparent from a young age. I didn't think anything truly psychic had ever happened to me. I'm not the seventh son of a seventh son, and I don't come from a family of gypsies. I'm not special. But with practice, I could become psychic. We are all psychic. We all have souls, and we can all listen to them.

Being psychic is about following your intuition, instinct, feelings, and perceptions, and allowing yourself to receive the information you need. So often I hear that students who are not visual want to be visual, even though they get clear messages in words. Others want to hear messages directly, but see vivid pictures. Some people do neither, but know things, and don't care that the message is accurate, because they want the bells and whistles that other people get. However you get information is the right way for you. Your only job is to find the way that is right for you, and honor it. As you grow and develop, your own method of receiving information can change and develop too.

Spiritual Gifts

Psychic abilities are a part of many healing traditions, from witchcraft to shamanism. In the Hindu traditions, those walking the mystic's path awaken these psychic abilities, called the siddhis. Although psychic skills are useful and demonstrate one's connection to the universe, such abilities are often considered liabilities because they are distractions on the spiritual path to enlightenment. Many get caught up in the power aspects of the siddhis and lose sight of enlightenment. In Western traditions, a practitioner must balance these psychic awakenings and the abilities that come with them while on the path, and in fact use such awakenings to demonstrate a higher spiritual reality.

In the ancient world, those gifted with naturally developed psychic abilities were guided into the mystical roles of priest/ess, seer, or healer, but in modern Western society, there are very few mystical roles to encourage those gifts. Reiki, in the medical and mystical sense, has become a "safe" avenue to explore healing and psychic ability. I know many people who would never explore witchcraft or ceremonial magick, but Reiki is okay because it is done in hospitals.

On the flip side of the coin, some practitioners come to Reiki feeling it is an aspect of the medical model, and have no interest in the mystical. And then, after the cleansing process of the first or subsequent attunements, strange things begin to happen. Intuition awakens. Clairaudience, clairvoyance, and clairsentience occur. Spirits speak. Auras come into fuzzy view.

Perhaps the Reiki attunement cleanses the third eye chakra, awakening psychic abilities. Perhaps it is the greater spiritual awareness of tuning in to the universal life force. Perhaps it is simply increased confidence when pursuing something wonderful. I don't know, but it does happen. And Reiki initiations are not the only way such things develop. They can come naturally. They can come with practice, meditation, and prayer. They can come with other magickal initiations and rituals. These spiritual gifts are the birthright of everyone, just like the universal life force.

Scanning

Scanning is a process that is usually taught in Reiki One (see chapter 3). Although I didn't learn it in traditional Usui Reiki, it seems to have a history in Japan. In either case, people don't seem to realize that scanning is a form of receiving information through psychic ability. Scanning consists of passing the hands slowly down the client's body, feeling the energy of the client's aura and chakras and interpreting this information to determine the level of health or imbalance in the person. Some attribute the energy sensitivity to the new Reiki attunement, but I've taught scanning in other healing magick classes that did not involve an attunement, and it seems that anyone can do scanning. Scanning is a psychic skill available to all.

Seeing Auras

Aura gazing is one of the most desired psychic abilities. People think psychics see a psychedelic panorama of colors surrounding them at all times, but in reality, most people who see auras know that the process is very subtle. It's like looking at the spaces in between, and is not always a bright and vivid experience.

I've found that if you are visually oriented, then you can learn to see auras. The important part of the exercise is to pick up information that can help you in your Reiki practice. Once when playing around with aura gazing with two psychic friends, we all learned something important. We each received our psychic information in a different way, but got very similar impressions. I was more visual and saw colors and images. My one friend saw different colors, but interpreted them the same way that I did. For one person, I saw bright yellow, but felt the person was nervous or stressed. My friend saw electric blue and came to the same conclusion. My other friend just "heard" the word yellow, through an internal voice, and felt nervous. The important thing was that we all connected to the information. The actual color doesn't matter as much, and can be subjective, regardless of what "aura photographers" will tell you. Such machines can be very helpful, but most interpret biofeedback information using common color interpretations. Auric energy is beyond the physical color spectrum.

Aura gazing is not for everyone. Don't get discouraged if the techniques given here don't work for you, and don't get hung up on wanting to have a certain experience. Find the techniques that work best to give you the most helpful information. I know many wonderful, powerful healing facilitators who don't use any psychic talents in their practice, but are still very effective work in their healing.

Exercise: Aura Gazing

To see an aura, start out with a taper candle against a white wall or background. Hang a white sheet if you don't have a white wall. Stare at the candle flame, and look for the shimmer around the flame. Then try to see a similar, but fainter, shimmer around the candle itself, as if you had drawn it down from the tip of the flame, to the candle, and eventually to the candle holder. When you get comfortable with the shimmer, look for a similar, but fainter, shimmer around other objects. Then try a plant or a person, something with living cellular tissue, against a white background.

When looking at a person, look for subtle breaks in the shimmering outline. They show where a person is losing energy and may have a pain, ache, or illness, or may have had a previous injury or illness that left an energetic mark.

Let your gaze go into an even softer focus while staring at the person. The shimmer will give way to an expansion of light. It too will be very faint, and if you focus on it too strongly, it might even disappear. You can almost catch it better with your eyes out of focus. The light will be diffuse at first, but you may see a sphere or egg of subtle light around the person. What color is the light? How do you feel or what do you think of when you see it? What is your first impression of it? Are there any darker spots that seem unhealthy? Where are they? Do you see anything else in the egg?

A lot of books will give you definitions for each color of the aura, but I've found that your first impression, your own personal interpretation, is the most important. There are many shades of colors. Sunshine or lemon yellow may indicate vitality, but pale yellow could be stress or toxification. If you don't like yellow, it will never indicate vitality for you. You might see orange or red in a vital aura. So go with your first impression.

Reiki Protection Shield

One function of the aura, regardless of your ability to see it or not, is protection. The aura is the field of protection and boundary. People with a weak or diffuse aura take on a lot of stuff from others and have no sense of personal space or boundary. An aura that is too rigid can have a brutish presence, repelling others from a space. A healthy aura is powerful and dynamic, yet soft and yielding when appropriate. A healthy aura is flexible and adaptable to any situation.

Mystical traditions teach people to program their aura with the intention of protecting and shielding themselves from physical harm as well as psychic harm from other people and entities. With the magick of Reiki, you can use the symbols to program your aura for protection and create an adaptable shield. I do this exercise daily, to create a sacred space around me that moves as I do.

Exercise: Protection Shield

Sit quietly and breathe deeply, getting into a meditative state. Imagine yourself in the center of a clear crystal egg or sphere. Draw Cho Ku Rei in front of you, in your mind's eye, as a shield of Reiki love. Then draw one to your right. Then imagine one being drawn behind you, and finally draw one to your left. Imprint them in the aura. Then draw Nin Giz Zida from your crown to root, and then Raku from your crown to the ground. You will be protected and centered, yet open.

Astral Travel and Distance Communication

Another psychic talent sought out by many is the ability to astral travel or remote view. It consists of sending your consciousness out to another place and perceiving that place with accuracy. Some practitioners can even make their presence known to others at the location they visit. Astral travel along the physical plane is sometimes called remote viewing, because there are physical markers that can be verified. Governments actually train psychic spies in this art. Other forms of such projection include shamanic journey and travel to the inner planes.

Most people who are interested in astral travel want to have an out-of-body experience and see the physical world. Again, expectations run high. Astral travel can be an amazingly vivid and physical experience for some, but not always. The important thing to consider is why do you want to do this, and what information will it give you? I often get very accurate information via astral travel, but don't have an intense experience. Students of mine have experienced an intense out-of-body sensation, but the information they got wasn't accurate.

To use Reiki to facilitate this process, start as if you were doing a distance Reiki session (see chapter 4). Instead of focusing on making a connection with a person via the Hon Sha Ze Sho Nen symbol, focus on a place. Imagine yourself stepping through the Distance symbol portal and traveling through a tunnel of light. Step out at the location you connected to, and imagine taking a look around. Use your intuition to determine shapes, colors, objects, and even people. What are your impressions? Don't expect anything, just let it occur.

When done, travel back through the tunnel of light. Erase the Distance symbol gateway and thank it. When you open your eyes, write down all your impressions, and if the location was a place you can visit, compare your impressions with reality to see how accurate you were. You will probably not be 100 percent correct, but every correct "hit" you get is a great feat. Your ability will improve as you practice.

Exercise: Phone Reiki

Try experimenting with sending Reiki to someone while talking to them on the phone. You can use Hon Sha Ze Sho Nen to make a magickal connection with them, but you can set it up like a combination of a psychic phone reading and a healing session.

Once you are connected with your recipient on the phone and have permission to send Reiki, draw or visualize Hon Sha Ze Sho Nen right over the phone. Think about the person as you chant "Hon Sha Ze Sho Nen" three times. You can feel the Reiki flow through the hand holding the phone to the recipient. The Reiki energy isn't literally flowing through the phone; it is flowing through your distance connection created by Hon Sha Ze Sho Nen, but the phone acts like a surrogate. You can use your intuition to do a scan, mentally visualizing the person and scanning their energy, since they are not physical present. Your Reiki/phone connection might make it easier to use your other psychic senses when speaking with the person. In some sessions, I just continue the conversation as I normally would, and let the recipient bring up any issues that need to be discussed. Other times, I use my intuition to guide the conversation, like an informal counseling session, bringing up whatever issues my intuitive abilities guide me to discuss.

Medical Intuition

Medical intuition is a psychic skill that combines visual, auditory, and clairsentient impressions to diagnose health and illness on the physical and energetic levels. It is practiced by witches, psychics, healers, and many Reiki practitioners. Some report that the skill develops or grows after a Reiki attunement, but this is not an absolute.

Exercise: Psychic Diagnosis

I learned medical intuition as a part of my witchcraft training, although we didn't call it that at the time. The basic technique consists of relaxing and getting into a meditative state. Once relaxed and in this meditative state, recite the name, the age, and the location of the residence of your intended "target." Ever since I received my Reiki attunements, I start the process like a distance Reiki session, creating a gateway to the recipient via Hon Sha Ze Sho Nen. This technique is similar to a distance Reiki treatment, though we will be extending the scanning techniques.

The recipient doesn't need to be physically present during the process. In fact, some practitioners can get accurate physical descriptions, including height, weight, hair color, and eye color, of people they have never met. But being able to get an accurate physical description is not really the point. The point is to make a diagnosis.

In your mind's eye, be aware of the target. You may see a person, or simply an outline of a person. Scan the image in your mind's eye, from head to feet, several times. Are there any points that catch your attention? If so, bring your attention to each one. What part of the body is there? What organs and body systems are present? Is it associated with a particular chakra? Is there a feeling or thought that seems to be attached to this area?

Gaze more closely at the area. Imagine going in deeper, getting more details and impressions. They might not be visual, but auditory or a sense of knowing. You can use the scanning technique to get tactile impressions using your hands. What are your impressions? What is wrong with that area? Is it connected to any other part of the body or any other imbalances? Continue to ask yourself these questions, and see where they lead.

Be aware that you might be struck not only by physical impressions, but emotional and mental ones as well. If they become overwhelming, simply ask to break the link with this person in a manner that is good and correct. Imagine Cho Ku Rei as a shield between you and the target. It will protect you. If you open your gateway connection using the distance techniques of Hon Sha Ze Sho Nen, you cannot be harmed by any of the recipient's energies since your connection is based on the Reiki energy and only flows one-way. You are only receiving psychic impressions through the connection, not taking on energetic imbalances. Even though you cannot be harmed with this technique, you could feel overwhelmed, so be gentle with yourself. Complete the session with detachment and don't worry about making a diagnosis for now. As you practice, your abilities will expand.

When done, send the recipient any Reiki symbols you feel would be of benefit, or do a Reiki distance treatment. Return from this level of meditation, closing the gateway between you and the recipient.

Psychic Surgery

The techniques of psychic surgery have become entwined with many Reiki Master classes, particularly in the Usui Tibetan traditions. Many misconceptions surround psychic surgery. One definition of it is a form of physical surgery, actually cutting and removing tissue without surgical instruments. Although I admit it's a possibility, I haven't seen such a technique performed in person. Some people have advertised such services, but it turned out to be a sham.

In Reiki, psychic surgery refers to something different. In Reiki, all things have an energetic root, and such psychic surgery removes the energetic root of illness. Without that energetic pattern, physical illnesses can collapse and be healed by the body's own natural systems much more easily. But it doesn't involve actual physical cutting on any level.

Although I learned psychic surgery techniques as a part of my Reiki Master apprenticeship, I later found the same techniques while studying various traditions of shamanism. Anthropologists have documented shamans performing such types of surgery, often using tubes to "suck" out the illness from a patient. In order to ensure that the energy would not be absorbed by the shaman, a rock, plant, or bug was placed in the shaman's mouth beforehand to be the receptacle of the unwanted energy. The shaman would spit out the substance and say the illness was sucked out. The anthropologists assumed that the "ignorant" tribal people thought the rock or insect was literally being sucked out of their own body, the source of the illness, and that the shamans were a fraud, tricking the clients. Little did they know that the tribal people were raised in this culture and knew the whole process and understood it in a way that the anthropologists could not.

The psychic surgery techniques found in the West, particularly in Western branches of Reiki, resemble techniques found in the Hawaiian shamanic tradition called Huna. Practitioners speculate that these techniques were added to Reiki at Mrs. Takata's Hawaiian school by one of her students. I've found other healers in non-Reiki traditions intuitively pulling out and releasing unwanted energies from clients, often pictured as stones, insects, serpents, leeches, or dark balls of oil, tar, or black light. Regardless of the origin, I think this process is universal to energy and spiritual healing.

The following is a simple version of these techniques, similar to what I learned. What is important to me is the interaction with the client, asking them questions and engaging them in the process of healing. That is the most important aspect of the healing process.

Step One

Discuss with the client what needs to be removed. It could be feelings from the past, relationships, obsessive thoughts, or memories—anything that needs to be released and healed. These usually indicate shadow aspects of the self, which aid in the creation of their unwanted reality or illness. Clients may have no idea of what needs to be released on the emotional or mental level, so let them describe their concerns in the best terms they can.

Step Two

Ask the client questions to provoke images, feelings, and qualities of the energy that is in need of removal. Questions could include the following:

- If it is within your body, where would it be?
- If it has a color, what would the color be?

- If it has a texture, what would it feel like?
- If it has a temperature, what would it feel like?
- It if makes a sound, what would it sound like?
- If it has a smell, what would it smell like?
- If it has a taste, what would it taste like?
- If it has a name, what would it be called?

Use the answers to these questions to build an image of the unwanted energy for both of you to work with.

Step Three

After creating this image and attaching it to the unwanted energy, ask the client if they can feel it, see it, or otherwise sense it within them.

Step Four

Prepare yourself by asking for higher guidance. Call in your healing and/or Reiki guides to be with you. Fill yourself with healing and protective energy. If you did not put the Power symbol in all your chakras and hands before the session, do so now.

Step Five

Imagine elongating your fingers by stretching your right-hand fingers out with your left hand, and vice versa. They may appear round and soft, or clawlike. (Other images may be needed, like scissor hands for cutting cords, or scalpel fingers for getting deep.)

Step Six

Through a combination of intent, movement, and visualization, imagine that you are reaching into the client and pulling/cutting/dissolving this harmful energy out of the body. Involve the client by touching them, so they know where you are and can feel the energy that needs to be released. Those who do psychic surgery above the body, without touch, leave the client feeling disconnected. I like to describe the process out loud to the client, to keep us both focused on the same image and intention. Tell the client to release or push the energy out. Use imagery consistent with the answers to their questions to create a shared, healing reality. This process may be done once or many times in a row, as you feel necessary.

At times, in this shamanic reality, the energy takes on a life and personality of its own, much like an individual entity or personality. Some practitioners report having to explain to the energy why it is being released from the body. If the energy appears to have a persona or intelligence, ask it for a message for the client. What is its purpose? Many energies are filled with harmful emotions such as fear, shame, and anger. If that is the case, tell the energetic entity that it is forgiven. Command it to go back to the light or return to its source, in love. By returning to the source, it will ultimately go back to the divine creator. Your healing spirit guides can help you banish these forces. Simply call upon them, out loud or silently, and ask them to remove the unwanted entity.

Step Seven

Take the harmful energy and dissolve it, releasing it in a manner that works for you.

- Use a combination of the Power symbol—Mental/Emotional symbol—Power symbol, three times each, and repeat the series three times to dissolve the energy.

- Visualize a violet flame burning up the energy.

- Send the energy out of the room, outdoors, and imagine it burning up.

- Ask your guides, deities, or angels to take the energy from you and transmute it.

- Command in the name of (your name for the creative spirit—God, Goddess, or Great Spirit) that the energy be banished and neutralized. Always remember to neutralize or transmute the energy before releasing it, so it does not attach to anyone else.

Step Eight

Repeat steps 1 through 7 for any other "surgery" points.

Step Nine

Cleanse and purify yourself and the client. First return your fingers (your etheric fingers) to their normal size and shape through touch and visualization. Then fill yourself with cleansing energy or violet light. Use protection symbols again. Finish the treatment and cleanse, sweep, and smooth the client's aura.

Psychic surgery techniques vary from practitioner to practitioner. You have probably done this before and not even known it since it seems so intuitive in healing work. The execution of psychic surgery can be outwardly very dramatic and ritualized, with a loud and commanding voice or broad sweeping motions, or it can be very internal and quiet, with simple, subtle movements and a confident intent. Everybody has a different style. It some ways, it's like play-acting with intention behind it. Remember this when feeling daunted by it, and keep your childlike perspective. Incorporate psychic surgery into your Reiki practice when you are comfortable with it and feel intuitively guided to do so.

Reiki Shamanism

As psychic surgery originated in the shamanic traditions, other Reiki practitioners have fused aspects of shamanic work and belief to Reiki, even creating Shamanic Reiki traditions. Shamanism is a word that come from the Siberian tribes of native people, but through a genetic link, also refers to the native people of North and South America. The word shaman typically refers to a tribal medicine man and healer, although the basic techniques of shamanism are found worldwide and differ from other practices of healing.

A shaman is one who acts as healer, religious leader, counselor, and doctor to a people. One of the main methods of healing is entering a trance state via meditation, drumming, dance, ritual, or psychedelic substances. After entering a trance state, the shaman contacts the spirit world, either bringing spiritual entities into the physical world to effect healing, or journeying to the spirit realm and bringing back information, knowledge, or power. Shamans not only enter the spirit realm, but can help guide others into this realm too, helping others with initiation rituals and vision quests. Shamans speak to the spirits of nature to learn about herbalism and stone healing. They speak with the powers of the elements, sky, and animals to ensure good weather for the growing season and good hunting for the tribe. Although the mythologies and beliefs behind the practice vary among tribes and cultures, the basic workings are found in Europe, Africa, the Middle East, and Asia. Modern shamanism, or core shamanism as it is now called, drawing from the core techniques, is finding its way into healing modalities, from avant-garde psychology to energy healing.

Besides psychic surgery, I've found two powerful shamanic techniques that I use in my Reiki practice. The first is to enter a trance state. If you have fast drumming music, all the better, since the beat helps enter an empowered shamanic trance state. Imagine yourself entering the body of the client, shrinking down low and traveling around the blood vessels, nerves, and other body parts, down to the cellular level. You can perceive things on a very physical level, feeling body parts, cells, or even molecules. Or you can view the "landscape" in a more symbolic way, traveling through underworld forests and jungles, crossing "rivers" of blood, and finding monsters of illness.

Through these techniques, you can literally find illness, physical or otherwise, and speak with its spirit and determine why it is present and what its purpose is. You can make deals and pacts with the sickness spirits or determine what they require to bring healing. Once you have completed your conversation with this spirit, and made any arrangements or gotten information, return the way you came and ground yourself back in the body. Then complete your session and speak to the client about what you found.

The second technique is exactly the same, but instead of you journeying into the body, through guided imagery, guide the client into his or her own body, to speak with the spirits of illness. Granted, this technique is not for everyone. The client may have no interest or aptitude for guided journey, but clients will surprise you. Many people whom I never thought would do this have done so, and I only pursued it initially because my intuition guided me.

Step One

Guide the client into a meditative state by counting backwards from twelve to one, encouraging them to relax their body, mind, and spirit.

Step Two

Tell your client to imagine their body getting smaller and smaller. With each breath the client becomes smaller, until they are microscopic. With them are any tools they need for the job. Tell them to look in their pockets and they will find their tools, such as material tools like picks, axes, swords, or torches, or metaphysical tools like crystals or herbs. Anything could be a tool, no matter how silly. Bubble gum, window cleaner, or a fan could be a tool in their pocket. The pockets can hold anything, of any size. Also with them will be a guide—a spirit, angel, loved one, or even a stuffed animal.

Step Three

Guide the client into entering the crown of the physical body. I often chant Sei He Ki, out loud or silently, to open the gateway. The client enters a tunnel and sees a distant light, leading them to the part of the body in need of healing. Ask the client, "Where is the light coming from?"

Step Four

Guide the client to go to that body part. Along the way they see the body parts. Encourage them to give love and light to the body along the way. If the client is a Reiki practitioner, tell them to do Reiki on the body parts or draw the symbols along the way.

Step Five

If the client gets lost or needs help, their guide will have the answer needed and point them in the right direction.

Step Six

Once the client reaches their destination, they find the spirit of illness. Encourage them to speak to it, to ask it what it wants, why is it here, and what can be done to heal it. Tell the client to listen with their heart. The guide may be needed to translate or act as an intermediary. The sickness spirit or guide may encourage healing through using the tools initially found in the pockets. Use them as guided.

Step Seven

If possible, tell the client to embrace and love the illness as a great teaching spirit. If the client is a Reiki practitioner, again have them do Reiki on the sickness spirit and offer it Reiki symbols. The sickness spirit may or may not dissipate into the ethers at this point.

Step Eight

When done, guide the client back through the body, radiating love and light.

Call upon your intuition and higher guidance when using any of these psychic and shamanic techniques in your magickal healing work.

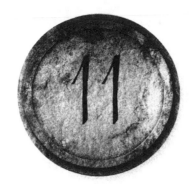

Crystal Reiki

The use of stones, minerals, and crystals in the arts of healing date back literally to the Stone Age. Evidence of such healing is found in the traditions of shamanism as well as in documents dating back to ancient Egypt, Sumer, and Greece, which list different stones and their metaphysical properties when carried or worn. These cultures all had vast traditions of magick, crafting talismans and charms from the stones and empowering them with divine blessings to catalyze their natural spiritual properties. Stone magick was one of the first types of magick.

The art of crystal healing found its way into the modern New Age movement and eventually into the healing traditions of Reiki. I'm not surprised, as the two systems are very complementary and compatible. Practitioners have created various traditions of crystal Reiki. In fact, the practice has become so prevalent, particularly at the Master levels, that I have found some students who think you can't practice Reiki without crystals. When learning the Usui history, they are told that Usui gave away quartz points and crystal balls to all his students. As far as I know, this isn't true. It goes back to the problem of people not identifying what they have added on to Reiki, and what is pure Reiki. You don't need anything to do Reiki other than an attunement, and some would even argue you don't need that. But crystals make wonderful helpers, particularly in Reiki. I love to use them both in my healing practice and personal life. I have more crystals than I have clothes.

Do Crystals Work?

Yes, crystals work. They don't affect everybody strongly or in the same way, but I have witnessed quite a number of remarkable changes in people using crystals and minerals. I use the word crystal for any mineral that has metaphysical properties, even if it is not a true crystal structure.

I used to think, "Big deal. They are pretty rocks. What can they really do?" Then I saw certain stones literally shift people's energy and patterns. Some crystals energize and awaken, while others help you meditate and relax. Some can get certain people almost high, while others can bring up repressed emotions and grief to be immediately healed.

The effects vary from person to person. If you are very grounded, very strong with the Earth energy, than crystals may not have an immediate dramatic effect. People would hand me stones and say, "Can't you feel the energy? It's amazing!" I must admit that no, I really couldn't feel much. A little, maybe, if I tried, but not what they were talking about. I am a very grounded person for the most part, and it took me a long time to understand the subtleties of stone magick. Even if the effect is psychosomatic (and I really believe it is not, since so many clients have no idea what each crystal is for), crystals are a powerful method of healing.

How Do Crystals Work?

Crystal healing works through the principles of vibration, another way to describe energy. Each mineral has a structure to it, often referred to as the crystalline structure. It is the basis of the chemical composition, the structure of the molecules. The "sacred" geometry inherent in these substances contains the principles.

Each chemical compound in the crystal gives it both physical and metaphysical properties. Physical properties include the color of the crystal and the shape in which it grew. The metaphysical properties often correspond with the color and shape, but are truly divined by working with the energy, the spirit of the crystal. Heart stones are often green and pink. Third eye stones are often purple.

When crystals are laid on the body, or carried in the pocket, they vibrate at a certain rate, based not only on their physical chemical structure, but on their more subtle energies, their spirit or life force. These vibrations are assimilated by the user, and slowly the properties of the vibrations are transferred to whomever is using the stone, bringing about healing or new awareness and abilities. To the metaphysician, everyone and everything is made of energy, of vibration, be it vibrating molecules or vibrating thoughts and emotions. Everything is energy.

Crystals 101

When teaching crystals, I describe their functioning much like a computer. Their structure records and remembers things, like computer memory, and they have the ability to speed up functions and do many things at once. Like a computer, they must be programmed. Whatever intention you put into the crystal determines what you get out of it.

Just like a computer, to maximize functioning, you must clean your crystal, removing any older, unwanted programs and random junk files. Since the crystal is like a spiritual version of the magnetic hard drive of your computer, every thought or feeling you have when holding it can be imprinting on the crystal. Those random programs and unwanted energies must be cleaned out.

Start by cleansing a crystal before you program it. You cleanse it by raising its vibration using techniques that remove unwanted energy. This banishes all unwanted programs and thoughts from the stone, without removing any of the healing energy. Try any one or a combination of the following techniques.

Smudge

Pass the stone through the smoke of a sacred cleansing herb or incense. Try sage, cedar, sweet grass, copal, frankincense/myrrh, lavender, cinnamon, cloves, juniper, or dragon's blood. Some burning herbs, although very magickal, are not protective or cleansing, so do some research before deviating from this list.

Sun

Keep the stone in direct sunlight for at least an hour to remove unwanted energies. Some stones, such as rose quartz, are sensitive to light and will fade with prolonged exposure to sunlight.

Flame

Pass the stones over a candle flame. Just be careful not to burn yourself. Don't hold the crystal in the flame, but above it at a comfortable distance. Imagine the energy of the flame consuming the unwanted programs.

Water

Soak your stones in clear spring or distilled water. You can hold them under running tap water, or, if you are really lucky to have one nearby, hold them in a running brook. The water carries away the unwanted programs and breaks them apart. Some crystals, like selenite, are water soluble and will dissolve, so always make sure your stone will not melt. Most crystals are fine in water, particularly anything in the quartz family—rose, citrine, amethyst, smoky, and strawberry quartz are quite safe to cleanse in water.

Salt

Bury your stones in a bowl of sea salt. Salt is a mineral that naturally absorbs the unwanted energies. Some people like to soak crystals in salt water, but long-term use is harsh to the stone both physically and energetically. I suggest using dry salt instead.

Earth

Bury your stones and ask the Earth to draw out unwanted energies. Keep them buried for anywhere from a day to a month. Just make sure you leave a marker so you know where to dig them up.

Prayer and Intention

Simply hold the stone in your hands. Ask in the name of the higher powers, whatever you choose to call them, that the stone be free from all harmful energy. I hold the stone up to my mouth and blow on it three times, blowing away the unwanted energy and transforming it with my intention.

Now you are ready to program your crystal. Hold it in one or both hands. Some people like to hold it to the third eye, while others prefer the heart. Do whatever your magickal intuition tells you to do. Then simply hold your program, your specific intention for the crystal, clearly in your mind, and using your will, imagine projecting that program into the crystal. Feel it move through your body, either out your hands or third eye, depending on which technique you chose, and then into the crystal. I put the following programs into my crystals, thinking the words in bold type. The additional text gives you information as to how this program works.

Act for the highest good. This empowers the crystal to work only for the highest and best healing good, and not force ego intentions on another.

Manifest all your powers as needed. This tells the stone to manifest the healing properties it has, as needed for the highest good, even if you are not consciously aware of them.

Activate/deactivate on command. The crystals will work with you, and activate and deactivate as needed. It sounds strange, but you can really tell the difference between an active and inactive crystal. This is a particularly powerful command for Reiki grids, which we will discuss later in this chapter. The crystals will also automatically deactivate if they are not for the highest good of the recipient.

Channel Reiki as needed. I then put all the Reiki symbols for the Usui Tibetan tradition into the stone, and any others I am intuitively guided to use. The stone will now channel Reiki energy as needed for the recipient.

Self-cleansing. You can program stones to help cleanse themselves of unwanted energies and programs. This doesn't mean you won't have to periodically cleanse your stones through other traditional methods, but it keeps you from having to do it each and every time you use them.

Programs are fixed for the highest good. This keeps these programs set in the crystal, so they cannot be removed by anyone unless it is for the highest good to do so. It's like pulling the record tab of an old cassette tape. You don't have to worry about anyone changing or erasing your programs accidentally.

You can also do specific crystal magick spells, programming a stone through Reiki and ritual to enact a specific change in your life. Experiment to see what works best for you.

Laying on Stones

In Reiki healing, crystals are usually incorporated into a hands-on session by laying the stones on the body. Although a lot of books and teachers gives rules about stone placement, there are no real rules. Most of it is an art and an act of following guidance. When placing stones, we often align stone color with chakra sites, but this is not a hard and fast rule. Until you get comfortable using stones and listening to their voices, and the voice of your guidance, try this list for each chakra.

Root	Garnet, ruby, red jasper, smoky quartz, red calcite
Belly	Carnelian, orange calcite, moonstone
Solar Plexus	Citrine, topaz, pyrite, yellow or golden calcite
Heart	Rose quartz, emerald, aventurine, malachite, tourmaline, green calcite
Throat	Blue lace agate, turquoise, lapis, azurite, blue calcite
Brow	Amethyst, purple flourite, lepidolite, sugalite
Crown	Clear quartz, opal, diamond, any clear or dazzling stone

Try placing one stone on each chakra and leave it there for a few minutes. As you become more familiar with the healing properties of these stones, you will use more creative healing layouts with more crystals in a greater variety of colors and patterns.

I like to do Reiki on an area first, and then place a stone there when my hand has been removed. That keeps the energy and healing strong throughout the body. Some people like to put the stone on first, and then do Reiki over the stone. As long as you don't apply pressure to the body or use jagged stones, that is fine.

When removing the stones, I imagine a string connecting the stone to the body. I imagine myself gently cutting the string, so the stone and body disconnect.

Reiki Crystal Grids

Crystal grids are a way to align crystals, usually quartz points, to intensify and magnify energy for manifestation or healing. In Reiki, the crystals are programmed to magnify Reiki energies for healing.

In a grid, crystals are arranged in a geometric structure to direct energy inward or outward, like a sacred mandala. The most popular shape, both in the crystal world and the Reiki world, is the six-pointed star, though each shape brings its own unique properties. I think the six-pointed star is associated with integration, balance, and the heart chakra, so it is a perfect shape to use in Reiki.

Reiki grids are usually taught in the more New Age versions of Reiki, from the Tibetan traditions on out, as part of the Master Practitioner or Master Teacher levels. Reiki crystal grids are used to send Reiki continuously to a recipient. In a Reiki session, distant or in person, you are limited to the time of the session. With a grid, the Reiki energy can continue to be sent even when the person who set it up is off doing other things. There are many grid techniques, including using the Antahkarana symbol as the grid pattern. I use the following symbol technique.

Step One

Take six quartz-crystal points of a similar size that you have already cleansed and charged, and place them on a hard surface where they will not be moved over a period of time. Arrange them like a six-pointed star, with the points pointing inward. If they are double-terminated, or double-pointed, you will intend that the energy flow inward as you do this.

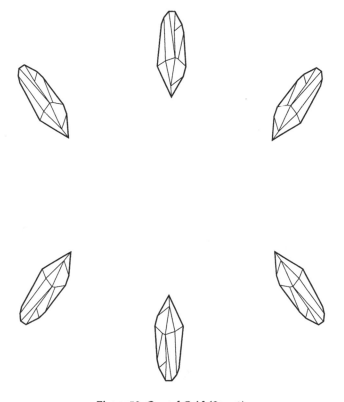

Figure 52: Crystal Grid (Step 1)

Step Two

In the center of the star, place something that will connect you to the person to whom you wish to send Reiki. It can be a photograph, a piece of jewelry, or a piece of paper with the person's name on it. You can have many recipients in the grid.

Step Three

Take a moment to center yourself, and say an evocation or prayer for divine guidance. Ask to send Reiki to this person, or people, for the highest good. Moving clockwise, activate the crystals in the first triangle by simply pointing to them and saying "Activate" silently or out loud. Do this three times around the triangle.

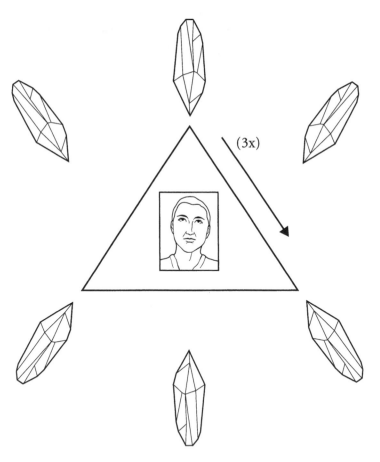

Figure 53: Crystal Grid (Steps 2 and 3)

Step Four

Continue with the second triangle. Activate each crystal, moving clockwise until you have gone around the triangle three times.

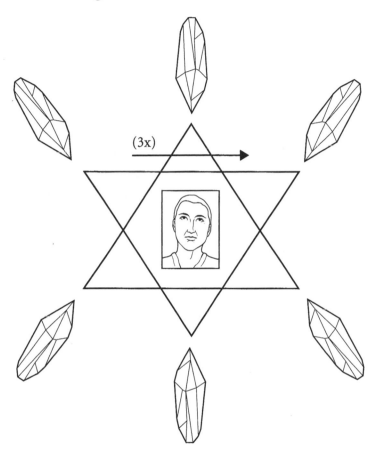

Figure 54: Crystal Grid (Step 4)

Step Five

Envision the center of the grid filling with Reiki light and going off to the ones in need. You can draw the Reiki symbols over the grid if you desire, to add to the intention of healing.

The Reiki grid can be activated and deactivated upon command. It will deactivate on its own when it is no longer for the highest good to send Reiki, when the person is "full," so to speak. So I like to reactivate it every day when using it. I make it a part of my morning devotional prayers. It's a powerful way to send healing when you cannot focus on the recipient.

Reiki and Jewelry

Practitioners of some Reiki traditions say that you shouldn't wear metal jewelry, such as rings, or other stones when doing Reiki. They believe that these substances impede the flow of Reiki energy. In my experience, that is not the case. I have found that if anything, they amplify and aid the process, as long as you have cleansed and programmed your jewelry. I treat all my jewelry like crystals, since metals are minerals with spiritual properties too.

I think if an authority figure tells us that something will impede us, then we will often believe the person and perceive ourselves as being impeded. But if an authority figure doesn't say anything, then we will not notice such blocks.

I encourage you to work with the spirit of the crystals and see how they change your own healing work, personally and professionally.

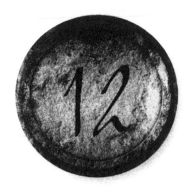

Reiki and Plant Magick

As Reiki is compatible with our allies from the mineral world, it is equally helpful with our green allies in the plant world. The magick of herbs and trees is powerful for healing and transformation. The first healers were the medicine folk who knew the herbs, medically and spiritually. These shamans and seers were the first ones to use their healing touch and work with the energy of the universe, via the Earth, Sun, Sky, and Moon. These hands-on healers were the first Reiki practitioners, in function with the energy, if not the current system. Modern Reiki amplifies the power of this magick.

I have found that using Reiki on anything amplifies its natural healing qualities. When we do Reiki on our food, to bless it, we bring out its healing qualities and minimize any impurities. When we do Reiki on our medicine, we enhance the healing qualities, to work in harmony with the universal good.

In witchcraft and other forms of earth magick, we charge, or bless, each component in our spells (the herbs, stones, oils, etc.) to consciously or unconsciously connect with its natural spirit and catalyze the spiritual properties of the substance. That's why, when people tell me they followed a spell from a book but have no experience doing ritual or working with these energies, I am not surprised to hear the spell didn't work. Just because you mix the right substances together in the right proportions doesn't mean you automatically get the desired result. Your spiritual awareness is the key ingredient to success. I know several witches who are Reiki-initiated and feel that Reiki has completely enhanced their earth magick and herbcraft, achieving results beyond their expectations. This has triggered a small movement of witches who take Reiki classes just to enhance their magick, but have no real interest, at least initially, in the tradition of Reiki.

Enhance Herbal Medicine

If you use herbs in your regular health regime, from herbal tea to supplements and even more intensive forms of herbal healing, you can empower your herbal remedies with the power of Reiki. Simply hold the herbs or herbal product in your hands, and let the Reiki flow. Or draw the Reiki symbols over it. I use Reiki on all herbs and even on all my food, blessing and empowering it. I use it on prepackaged herbal teas, teas I blend myself, tinctures, and the spice rack. If you pick your own herbs, vegetables, or fruit, do Reiki on the food as you pick, but also on the plant you leave behind, so it too can heal and produce more healthy food.

Aromatherapy

Aromatherapy is the art and science of using scent to change consciousness, usually through the medium of essential oils extracted from flowers and plants. The use of magickal scents is an ancient practice, and working with the spiritual properties of plants is an important, yet often neglected aspect of aromatherapy work.

Magickal practitioners use oils both for anointing the person and for anointing ritual objects, charms, and, most often, candles. If you use Reiki with candle magick, you can anoint the candle with an appropriate oil that matches your intention magickally. You can also do Reiki on an oil and wear it to bring those qualities and intentions into your life.

Flower Essences

Flower essences are vibrational remedies made from very dilute solutions of flowers in water, preserved in a small amount of a stabilizer, such as brandy or vinegar. With the word essence in the name, many people confuse flower essences with essential oils used in aromatherapy. But while essential oils contain very concentrated forms of natural plant chemicals, flower essences are very dilute medicines with only trace amounts of plant chemicals. They are even more dilute than homeopathic remedies. In modern times, they were originally created by a homeopathist named Dr. Edward Bach, and his line of essences, called Bach Flower Remedies, is available commercially through most health food stores.

If flower essences have little to no chemical content, then how do they work? Much like Reiki, flower essences are an energy medicine. They work on an energetic vibrational level and often don't have a strong physical effect, but focus on the mental, emotional, and spiritual levels of a person, creating a change in consciousness that will bring healing on all levels.

When you make a flower essence, you bring the spiritual powers of that plant into your body for healing. Each flower carries the energetic signature of its unique properties, demonstrated by its shape, colors, growth pattern, and folklore. These factors tell us what healing properties are embodied in the flower's energetic medicine. Some signatures are obvious. Roses are associated with the heart and love. When you take rose flower essence, you open your heart to love and remove the blocks that prevent you from experiencing or expressing love. It's not a magick pill that makes all blocks go away, but an energetic aid to help you work through those issues.

When I first began working with Reiki, my healing process brought up issues of anger and unresolved guilt. I was having liver problems, and through studying body symbolism and energy healing, and through my own meditations, I learned that the liver stores fear and anger. I continued to do Reiki, and it helped, but it didn't resolve the problem.

At a friend's recommendation, I decided to see a flower essence consultant, who immediately put me on flower essences made from herbs that are used to treat liver disease. Spiritually, these liver-healing herbs, such as milk thistle, are used to heal anger and fear, the spiritual roots of liver illness.

I was given a bottle of a variety of flower essences mixed together. I took three drops of the mixture, three times a day. Before I took the essence, I did Reiki on the bottle. I then would do a mini self-treatment.

The Reiki brought up unresolved feelings that I didn't know I had. I thought the essence would make them go away like magick, but it didn't. Within three days, I found myself expressing my anger to a superior at a new job I was starting. Normally, I would have gotten angry, swallowed it, and continued on in an unhappy situation. But this time, I expressed my anger. It was strong, but healthy. I wasn't happy about my reaction at first, though. I was mad at the essences for "making" me angry. They didn't make me angry—they brought my anger up to the surface to be expressed and healed. The combination of Reiki and flower essences helped me heal on the deepest level and resolve a lot of long-standing issues.

Even though many brands of flower essences are available commercially, I really encourage people to make their own essences and build their own magickal relationship with the plant world. Making essences is a very simple process, although some practitioners make it overly complicated. I have a folk-magick witchcraft background and apply the same simple spirit to my flower-essence making.

I am very ritualistic in my essence making. I go out to the flowering plant and meditate with it. I ask the plant for permission to make the essence and ask for information about its healing properties. Some people have psychic experiences with the plants, where the plant's spirit speaks to them, grants visions, or takes them on a spirit journey, but most people do not have such experiences. Whether you do or not is not indicative of the strength of the essence you are making.

Then place a clear glass bowl or quartz-crystal bowl (not lead crystal) near the flower on the ground on a sunny day, preferably in the morning. Fill it with water, either spring water or distilled water. I prefer spring water. Pick a few flowers and place them in the bowl. If the flowers are endangered, you can simply put the bowl of water beneath the flower, without cutting or picking the flower, so it can mature and go to seed. The energy of the flower will still go into the water, because the water is in the plant's energy field. Technically, you don't have to pick any flowers to make the flower essence, but most practitioners do.

You can incorporate Reiki into the process by drawing any symbols you want over the bowl and flowers. I use the Tibetan Master symbol, Usui Master symbol, Power symbol, Mental/Emotional symbol, Distance symbol, Nin Giz Zida, and sometimes Mer Ka Fa Ka Lish Ma and Zonar in various combinations, following my intuition. There is not one perfect and correct combination of symbols for all flower essences. Technically, the symbols are not required to make an essence, but add to and amplify the essence's natural healing properties. Let the bowl sit out in the sun for at least two hours. If it is cloudy, keep it out for at least four hours. This isn't a hard and fast rule. I often leave my essences out all day and all night. I like to make them at the full Moon and leave them in the sun all day and the under the Moon all night, collecting them at dawn.

When you feel the essence is "done," it is time to bottle it. Do the Reiki symbols over the essence again before bottling, to stabilize the healing vibration. The first bottling is called the mother essence. When you bottle the original water, strain the flowers out through an unbleached coffee filter, or simply pick the flowers out gently. Bottle the essence in a dark-colored bottle with one-fourth preservative by volume. Traditional preservatives are 80 proof or higher alcohol, such as brandy or vodka, which lasts the longest and prevents the solution from going rancid. If you prefer, you can use a nonalcoholic preservative, such as apple cider vinegar. It doesn't last as long, only a few years, as opposed to the potentially unlimited shelf life of vodka. Other essence makers use a vegetable glycerin or red shiso preservative. Once you bottle your mother essence with preservative, label and date it. I also shake it and do hands-on Reiki on it.

Then, when you want to use your essence, you will create weaker dilutions that have a stronger energetic effect. Flower remedies become more potent as they are diluted. Get a smaller bottle, such as a half-ounce dark glass dropper bottle, and mix a solution of 75 percent pure water and 25 percent preservative. Place five to ten drops of mother essence into the new bottle, and label it the stock bottle. Most retailers sell essences that are at this level of potency. The stock level of dilution often works on more of a physical level.

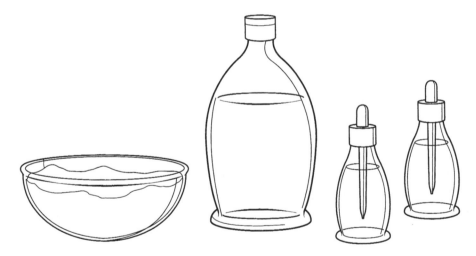

Figure 55: Essence Bowl, Mother Essence, Stock Bottle, and Dosage Bottle

To take an essence for the mental or emotional level, take one to five drops from the stock bottle and place into another bottle of 75 percent pure water and 25 percent preservative. You can mix several essences together at this level of potency for a specific intention. This is the dosage level of flower essences and is what flower essence consultants give out. Before I give an essence to a client, I do Reiki on it and hold it to my heart, asking that it be used for the highest healing good.

Plant Spirit Medicine

Plant spirit medicine is a relatively new term that describes the traditional practice of shamanic healing through partnership with the spirit of a healing plant. I feel that it is the root of all other herbal healing, from medicinal uses to aromatherapy and flower essences. All magickal healing consists of bringing all aspects of yourself into balance and alignment, and often it takes a partnership with another spirit energy to aid this process. Shamans know that the spirit of plants, animals, and minerals, as well as the energy of the universal life force, can act as "medicine" to us.

A shamanic practitioner will enter a trance and speak with spirits and guides, but will often ally himself or herself with the spirits of plants. Each plant has a specific range of powers in alignment with its personality, much like its flower essence signature. The shaman can call upon the plant spirit to bring its medicine to a client. Sometimes that involves taking a medicinal, homeopathic, or vibrational remedy of the plant. Other times, the exchange is purely energetic. The results can be very powerful.

One way to incorporate plant spirit medicine into a Reiki practice is to cultivate a relationship with the plant spirit guides, much like one might cultivate a relationship with Reiki spirit guides, angels, or ascended masters. Pick a few herbs with which you feel a connection, and learn all you can about them. If you can, meditate next to the physical plant. If it's not available in your area or at that time, meditate while thinking about the plant, visualizing it and silently chanting its name to make a connection to its spirit. Then ask permission to call upon it in healing.

Then, in your next healing session, if you feel intuitively that the plant's medicine could be of help, evoke the plant spirit and ask it to bring its medicine to the client. Deeper levels of shamanic work involve the practitioner going into a shamanic state of consciousness, projecting to the shamanic underworld or upper world, and bringing back the plant spirit medicine, and then blowing it into the client. But sometimes a simple evocation and prayer is all that is needed.

In the context of Reiki, I may invite the plant spirit medicine into the attunement process for a healing attunement, blowing the medicine in with the influx of Reiki symbols. You can even do mini Reiki/plant attunements. I draw Cho Ku Rei, then Iava—for nature connections—and then invite the plant spirit in. I close the process with Cho Ku Rei. The blended effects can be quite profound and immediate. For some, it is as if they have physically been taking the herb for months. Others feel no physical effect, but this healing technique manifests the spiritual healing properties of the plant in the person.

Herbal Charm Magick

Herbal magick is the first place I was introduced to the power of the plant world. I learned the art of brewing magickal potions and making herbal charms as part of my witchcraft training. As each herb has a healing vibration, a healing spiritual quality, it also has a magickal quality that is in alignment with that healing energy. (See appendix 2 for more information on the magickal and spiritual properties of plants.) Magickal herbs are divided into the basic categories of magick, including love, prosperity, protection, "curse" breaking, healing, health, knowledge, creativity, fertility, psychic awareness, and spiritual development.

Herbal magick works much the same way as candle magick. All forms of folk magick involve natural tools. The tools act as both vessels for the magickal intention and as spiritual partners for the working. The magician or witch must interact with them on an energetic level, catalyzing and activating the inherent magickal properties of the substance. The most common way of doing this is through touch.

Use the following formulas or make your own from your own magickal research and experience, based on the intent you wish to create. Hold each herb in your hands and let the Reiki flow. Think about the intent, and use your ability to speak, visualize, and intend to catalyze the herb, as if you were partnering and praying with the spirit of the plant. Do this for each ingredient. You can even combine this with crystal and metal magick, adding such things to the mix. Use whatever Reiki symbols you are guided to use, by drawing them and chanting their names over the mixture. Then carry the herbs in a small, colored pouch, choosing the color based on the magickal color correspondences. (See appendix 3 for color associations.) Here are some examples.

Protection Charm

    1 tablespoon vervain

    1 tablespoon patchouli

    1 tablespoon nettles

    5 hawthorn berries, rowan berries, or rose hips

Carry in a red or black bag.

Psychic Development Charm

    1 tablespoon lavender

    1 tablespoon mugwort

    1 tablespoon star anise

    1 tablespoon lemon peel

    1 tablespoon white yarrow

Carry in a purple, lavender, or white bag. You can sleep with it under your pillow for psychic dreams.

Fertility Charm

    1 tablespoon lady's mantle

    1 tablespoon basil

    1 tablespoon red clover

    1 tablespoon red raspberry

    1 tablespoon motherwort

    1 tablespoon watermelon seeds or rind

    3 tablespoons oats, corn, or any other grain

Carry in a green or red bag.

Part of "good" magick is the concept of the highest good, harming none. Most witches put this intent into all their spell work. It would be better for a spell to fail than bring harm. When empowering the tools with Reiki, you are reemphasizing the highest good, the higher will or universal life force's will, rather than pure ego. Through this, you can learn to partner and identify with the highest forces, through love and trust.

Reiki in the Garden

Use Reiki in every stage of gardening. Reiki the soil you are going to use by placing your hands on the soil and letting the Reiki flow, or by drawing Reiki symbols over the soil and activating them through chanting their names three times each. Reiki the plants and seeds when you put them into the soil. Reiki your fertilizer, and depending on your water source, Reiki the water you use to nourish it if that's practical. Visualize the symbols in the water spraying from the house. When you harvest, Reiki what you harvest, but also Reiki the remaining plant, to make an exchange, for it is giving you medicine, food, and/or beauty. I feel very strongly about exchange with the plant world—if we can take from it, we can give back to it as well. Unlike some physical offerings, such as food, coins, or candles, offerings of your time and healing energy can be the greatest gift to the garden and its spirits.

Earth Healing Reiki

I feel that healing the Earth with Reiki is a tremendous part of our spiritual practice in the world at this time, although it is not the most traditional way of working with the plant kingdom. The Earth is going through tremendous changes on all levels, and I believe that the great influx of Reiki is a part of that healing process. When we seek to heal the Earth, we can do many things.

When we seek to heal the Earth, we can bring healing on a multitude of levels. Most mystics believe that we are all connected. If we change and improve ourselves, we improve the overall energy of Mother Earth. It's a form of sympathetic magick.

When we heal ourselves, using Reiki or any tool at our disposal, from crystals to conventional psychology, we are sympathetically healing the world. We are all hooked into a greater human or earthly consciousness grid, and its energy is the overall vibration of everyone's collective thoughts and feelings. If you improve your own energy, your own vibration, then you help increase the overall consciousness. By helping others heal, you help the world heal.

Sympathetic magick is the act of performing one action, usually ritualistically, to symbolize a larger change you desire. The stereotype of the Voodoo doll is an act of sympathetic magick. Voodoo is perhaps the only spiritual path more maligned than witchcraft. In many traditions, the act sticking a pin into a poppet or doll that resembles another is done to stimulate healing in that area. Rain dances are another form of sympathetic magick. In some rain ceremonies, the last remaining precious water is spilled onto the earth ritualistically, to create a greater rain from the heavens.

Even the witches dancing around on their brooms in old Europe is an act of sympathetic magick. They were not trying to fly. They were jumping high with symbols of fertility (brooms) to make the crops grow tall. The higher they jumped, the higher the crops would grow. Not until this image was mixed with the legends of the witch's flying ointment, a psychotropic substance used as an aid in astral travel or shamanic "flying," did we have the legend of the witch flying on a broomstick.

Doing distance Reiki on a doll, pillow, photograph, or piece of paper with a name on it is an act of sympathetic magick. The energy of your symbolic actions is transferred to the recipient of the Reiki treatment.

Another important component in Earth healing is your physical behavior as a consumer in this world. We can do all the energy healing we want, but if we continue to run rampant through our natural resources with no thought to the future, then energy healing will not do us any good. Many New Age people feel that energy work and consciousness change is going to "zap" us into another dimension free of pollution, synthetics, and waste. As a fairly grounded, Earth-centered witch, that doesn't make sense to me. We are on the physical plane to learn about the physical plane. Even if we increase our level of consciousness, we will still need to deal with the mess we have collectively made. The first step is living in a more holistic manner. We each must decide what steps are most appropriate for ourselves and our families. If you haven't already done so, start thinking about living green, conservation, recycling, environmentalism, and organic food. Many spiritual teachers believe the Earth is capable of healing herself, but we have to stop causing damage and change our way of living with the Earth.

Reiki Earth healing can be as simple as laying your hands on the ground and asking the Reiki to flow. You can do group Reiki rituals with others, all laying hands on the world. I do distance Reiki healing to trouble spots in the world, such as centers of natural disasters or political unrest. In meditation, I simply say, "I ask to connect to Mother Earth. Mother Earth, is there any place you would like me to send Reiki to? Is there any work you would like me to do today?" Then I listen and see what comes to mind. Sometimes I am guided to send Reiki to a place that isn't even in the news, but I do it anyway. Sometimes it shows up later as a trouble spot, and other times it doesn't. Perhaps the

Reiki healed some situations completely, and thus they were never brought to the world's greater attention.

My favorite form of Reiki healing is one I learned from those in the Shamballa tradition. The founder of Shamballa, Hari Das Melchizedek, is heavily involved in Earth healing. This is my variation of a technique used by Shamballa practitioners and light workers.

Exercise: Earth Healing Grid

Start by arranging a Reiki grid, as described in chapter 11, with six quartz points. Have the points facing out. Arrange the grid on the Earth, at a place you feel guided to heal, particularly for energy, environmental, or spiritual healing.

State the following: "I ask to connect to Mother Earth and Father Sky. I ask to connect to Pan, to the devas and nature spirits of this place. I ask permission to do Earth healing here, for the highest good, harming none." Wait for an affirmative or negative response, as you would during a distance healing. Don't assume that you will always get a yes. Sometimes you will not, for reasons that are serving a higher good, even though it doesn't seem like it from our limited perspective.

If you receive a positive response, activate the two triangles of the six-pointed star. Feel them fill with light, and say: "I call upon the highest Reiki spirit guides and masters. I call upon the angels and archangels. Give me a pillar of healing Reiki light from the universal source, through this grid and into Mother Earth, for the highest good." Visualize a continuous beam of light coming down from the sky into the grid, empowering the crystals, and then diving down into Mother Earth.

Place any of the Reiki healing symbols you feel guided to use in the center of the star, and feel their energy not only pulse downward to the core of Mother Earth, but outward, through the points, in radiating waves of healing energy across the land. I recommend all the traditional Usui and Tibetan symbols, as well as Zonar, Mara/Rama, Iava, and Mer Ka Fa Ka Lish Ma. You may even "receive" symbols intuitively from the Earth that she wishes you to use in this task.

You can let the grid "run" for several minutes, up to several hours, as your intuition guides you. You can come back as often as you want, and repeat the symbols or put different ones in the grid. You don't necessarily have to be outside to do this, either. You can do it inside, placing the points inward, and placing a picture or symbols of the place in need of healing in the center, like a traditional Reiki grid. You can put a small globe or picture of the Earth in the center of your grid.

When done, deactivate the grid by asking the guides, masters, angels, and archangels to ground the pillar of light into the Earth for the highest good. Then ask the crystals to deactivate, one by one. Thank Mother Earth, Father Sky, Pan, and the nature spirits and devas. Finally, dismantle the grid itself.

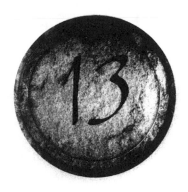

The Future of Reiki

Where is Reiki going? Where has it been? These two questions have no certain answers. The past of Reiki is shrouded in myth, with tales of ancient Tibet, China, India, Egypt, and Atlantis. We can't even seem to agree on the facts from modern Japan. Where is Reiki going? It's branching out in a million different directions and traditions, each as different as the practitioner and teacher using it. The process reminds me a lot of the eclectic traditions of paganism, witchcraft, and ceremonial magick, each with a variety of beliefs, practices, and traditions.

I started this path of exploring the "new" avenues of Reiki because I felt something was lacking in traditional Usui Reiki. The more I spoke with other practitioners, the more I heard those same sentiments echoed back to me. Usui Reiki is complete as a system in itself, but still, I wondered if there was some truth to these "fringe" ideas of ancient Reiki. That is why I explored and trained in the other branches of Reiki. I've found things I like and techniques that are useful, and I've shuddered at some of the spiritual "laws" I've been given by power-hungry practitioners who seek to control others and build followers.

The more I studied, the more I realized it all took me back to the heart of my spiritual truth—magick, responsibility, and service. To me, there is no difference in the truth of the witch or mage and that of the Reiki Master. The only perceived differences are the execution and window dressing.

Reiki Syndromes

Some of the things I hope to discourage are the unhealthy Reiki "syndromes" cropping up among those in "newer" traditions, who often lack the metaphysical understanding of their practice and spout lines learned by others, without really understanding their meaning and implication. Usually the teacher also lacked understanding and passed on only what he or she knew to be true.

The first syndrome is "My Reiki is better than your Reiki." This one is running rampant, I'm afraid, but many people don't even realize they have it. Practitioners from certain traditions will say that their form of Reiki is more intense, powerful, healing, loving, etc., than another tradition, in order to entice you to study it. Their tradition may have wonderful benefits and may differ greatly from the other traditions, but just because something is different doesn't necessarily mean it is better. The tradition may have better training and more experienced teachers, or the attunement itself may improve your ability to perceive the energy or personally bring in greater amounts of energy than you did previously. But with energy from the universal life force, we are all drinking from the same pool of water. You may like your spot better. It may have nice shade and pretty flowers, but the water is the same. Reiki is Reiki. The ways in which it manifests and the philosophies others attach to it may be more appealing to you, but please don't berate what others are perfectly happy using. We don't all have to match.

When I took my Shamballa training, many Shamballa Reiki Master-Teachers were former Usui Reiki teachers and were encouraged to give up teaching "regular" Reiki, because Shamballa was supposedly far superior and of a higher vibration. My Reiki practice changed completely for the better after my Shamballa attunements, and I started to attract the type of clients I wanted to work with, on the emotional rather than physical level, but I couldn't conceive of giving up Usui Tibetan Reiki. I was taught Shamballa with ascended masters, Atlantis, and angels. I like those concepts and energies, but they will not resonate with everyone. They are what was right for me at the time, to continue my path, but I can't conceive of having started there, and I can't see most people starting there.

My father took traditional Reiki, but would have walked out of a Shamballa class. I continue to teach traditional Reiki for people like my father. The "new" Shamballa energy is still with me, and I'm sure some of it is passed during my "regular" attunements if it is for the highest good of that person. It reminds me that I am not in control—the divine is.

The second prevalent Reiki syndrome is "I have hidden knowledge." I must admit, I succumbed at one point to this syndrome. For Reiki, it usually revolves around the symbols. I felt that Usui Reiki was missing some critical symbols. If I had knowledge of them, I would have the missing piece and everything would be clear in my life. I had no such luck, but I tried. I took many different classes and read many different books, seeking more and more symbols, in the hope that some tradition or teacher had the knowledge I sought. I love working with symbols, but in the end, I realized that they are only a tool. They won't make the Reiki, or my life, any better by themselves. They can't do anything more than I already can through intent and by laying my hands and letting the Reiki flow. There is no way to get "all" the symbols. But we try, and people perpetuate the syndrome by saying they have the new symbols. I will tell you that the more symbols I studied, the more silly they became and the less like Reiki it all felt. I have a large set of symbols that I like to use in my healing, but they are not my primary focus. Love, service, and magick are my focus.

One of the reasons I studied Shamballa was the promise of 352 symbols leading to the source. What I really liked about it in the end was that after the fourth attunement, you are "intuitively" attuned to all 352 symbols, and they will manifest consciously and unconsciously as needed. The entire collection is said to be comprised of these 352 symbols, but I'm sure there are more than that in use by people in various Reiki traditions. I prefer to think of it as 352 levels of energy, with a variety of geometric expressions. I think that no matter what your tradition, if you intuitively are called to use a "new" symbol and name, then do it. Let the Reiki guide you. Again, we are all connected to the same pool of energy, with access to the same symbols.

The third syndrome is "We must keep Reiki pure." Those afflicted with this one don't even want to talk about changing, adapting, or adding to Reiki. If you can't prove that Dr. Usui, Hayashi, or Takata did it, then don't do it. They are the purity police. Some even discount Hayashi and Takata, and seek a purely Japanese lineage without the "taint" of the West.

While I believe that, as a good teacher, you should disclose what is traditional Reiki and what has been added to it, I really feel that if something doesn't adapt and change with the needs of the people it serves, it dies out. I believe in personal freedom for teachers and students to use what works for them, but that they should be clear in their practice. A lot of concepts in Western Reiki are not Japanese, such as chakras, but they are very useful in Reiki. Such ideas blend harmoniously, at least in my practice. Witchcraft and ceremonial magick were forced to borrow concepts from Eastern and Western magickal traditions because many of the concepts and names were lost in the witchcraft persecutions of Europe.

The purity police are afraid of Reiki becoming ridiculous with so many New Age add-ons, and they have a point. In fact, their fears have been justified in some quarters, but if such things work for a person, then they work. Those seeking purity and wanting to establish scientific credibility follow the more medical models of Reiki, and will often not see eye to eye with the more mystical practitioners in the community. But there is room for both. We all need the freedom to do what works. If, in training, we are educated about what is and is not traditional Reiki, then it becomes less of a problem.

Reiki Fallacies

As the Reiki syndromes have crept up on us, so has a lot of false information about how Reiki works. The bottom line is that it is the universal life force, directed by higher consciousness. We are not in control of it. It can do no harm. If you keep these thoughts in mind, you can debunk most Reiki fallacies.

As I recounted in chapter 3, one of my first experiences with Reiki was after my level one class. I did Reiki on my mother, who experienced pain as part of her healing crisis. When we went to the doctor, the nurse said, "Oh, we don't know much about Reiki. You could have done more harm than good with it." If I had really understood the Reiki principles, I would have realized that it was just the nurse's fear speaking. At the time, few in the medical field knew anything about Reiki, but that seems to be changing. Now, many medical organizations have Reiki clinics run by nurses and other healthcare professionals!

Reiki, like most kinds of natural medicine, is self-adjusting. It knows when to warm, when to cool, when to relax, and when to tighten, on all levels. You don't have to worry about it. Just do Reiki. It reminds me of self-adjusting plant medicines such as yarrow and Solomon's seal. Yarrow works on the blood. If you need the blood thickened, it thickens it. If you need the blood thinned, it thins it. How does it know what you need? It just does. That is the living life force of the plant, not just the active ingredients, at work. Likewise, Solomon's seal root can be used on tendons and ligaments. If they are too loose, it tightens them. If they are too tight, it loosens them. It adjusts to bring you back into balance, just like Reiki.

When people tell me these fallacies, I always ask, "Have you found that to be true?" Most times the answer is no. If the answer is yes, I usually tell the person I haven't found that to be true, and the next time they try it, some report that their previous "fact" now turns out to be untrue for them as well. Perhaps it is all a matter of perception. If I have few limits for myself, I experience few limits. If I take on a lot of limited programming from others, I experience a lot of limits.

Since Reiki works for the highest good, it will not inhibit the effects of medicines if they are for your highest good. The highest consciousness is not biased against pharmaceuticals. If a medication is working for your highest good, it will keep working. People say all sorts of crazy things, like Reiki neutralizes medicines, or slows them down or burns them out of the system quickly, like a toxin. If it is for the highest good for a medication to be removed, it may, but in my experience, it hasn't.

Reiki will not awaken a patient under anesthesia during surgery. Why would it? Most people in my Reiki sessions come in awake and then zone out or fall asleep on the table. Reiki works for the highest good, and waking up on the operating table with a surgeon over you would probably not be for the highest good.

Likewise, Reiki will not sedate you if you receive a distance treatment while operating heavy machinery. Some traditions like for the recipient of the distance treatment to meditate or become more receptive and introspective during the session. I agree that it can add to the experience, but when certain teachers claim that distance Reiki must be done that way, I disagree. They claim that if a person receives Reiki healing while driving or operating other machinery, that they will become sedated, shocked, or so blissful that an accident will occur. I learned that Reiki works for the highest good, so if such danger would be the result, then the higher consciousness will regulate the energy or delay it until a more appropriate time.

Reiki, as a healing force, will not heal and encourage disease in the body. Some people say to avoid doing Reiki on tumors or viral infections, because it heals and strengthens the disease. Not true. Reiki works for the highest healing good, and will often precipitate a healing crisis so the recipient can fully understand what purpose the illness is serving. The healing crisis can be a traumatic emotional, mental, or physical release, and because of this, many people shy away from doing Reiki directly on an injury, infection, or tumor to tone down the intensity, but not because they are "feeding" the illness.

Growing with Reiki

As with any spiritual pursuit, the techniques may remain the same, but your experiences will deepen with practice. Though technically not a religion or even a formal spiritual practice, Reiki has become precisely that for many people. It acts as a foundation for spiritual and magickal awareness. Reiki opens a door for many people, in a world of great spiritual possibility.

If your experiences with Reiki start to change over time, don't be alarmed. That can be a natural part of the process. Likewise, if your experiences remain the same, that is not indicative of growth, but you may experience many other types of changes in your life. Your growth may simply not need to be reflected in your Reiki practice.

The biggest change I've noticed in my own practice is the intensity level of the Reiki energy. You might expect the energy flowing from a Reiki "professional" to become more and more intense, but in my self-treatments, it has become the opposite. Often I don't feel it. One practitioner explained it to me as a matter of vibration. She said that Reiki increases your vibration. When you are at a "lower," or less healthy, vibration, the Reiki can be felt intensely. As your everyday vibration begins to match the level of energy you bring through, by becoming healthier and more in balance, you don't feel the difference as much. I'm not sure if she is right, but it made sense to me at the time. When I am out of balance or have not been taking care of myself, I feel the energy more. And when I personally don't feel much in my self-treatments, my clients still feel it intensely, because they are not necessarily at the same vibration. Also, when I receive Reiki from others, I can feel it is different because I am not at their vibration. One type of vibration is not necessarily better or worse, it's just different.

The lack of intensity I felt during self-treatments was one reason I sought out other attunements in other traditions. I noticed a "jump" in energy when I studied another tradition, which led me to believe that these traditions were better than what I had learned. I think that each new attunement was just another opportunity to connect with Reiki on a deeper level and clear out even more of my personal psychic closet that inhibited me from fully flowing with Reiki. But I soon realized that the new attunements were not dramatically increasing the amount of energy I could channel. I didn't get the same "jump" in the energy level I was channeling during self-treatments. My ability to channel Reiki energy gradually rose with my regular practice of Reiki, but now I was channeling all the energy I was capable of channeling at the time.

Everyone is different, and can channel a different level or quality of energy. The energy can change over time and with practice. The energy can also change with different attunements from different traditions. Every tradition is slightly different, bringing the energy through different symbols and with different qualities. Don't confuse different with better. All you really need is your first attunement to Reiki to begin your journey.

I have found that working through doubt is a big part of the Reiki practice, as well as trusting in my experience, my previous experiences, and the universe. You might not think so by my outward appearance as a New Age, witchcraft, astrological crystal healer, but I'm pretty grounded, and at times I would think, "Is this even really working? Is this real? Have I convinced myself of something that isn't there?" It's easy to distrust the process because Reiki is so simple in essence. I figured there had to be a catch. By learning to detach and trust, I based my beliefs on my previous direct experiences of healing. Detachment and experience are the greatest teachers.

As a mystic, I have noticed that my personal ability to receive information or have a mystical experience while giving a Reiki treatment changes in phases. At times, I have had truly visionary experiences while giving Reiki. I've seen auras, chakras, and unhealthy energy forms during healing sessions. I've spoken with spirit guides and angels, and given their messages to my clients. But at other times, I have experienced nothing—no spirits, no lights, no messages. I would be thinking about my house chores, grocery list, work to-do list, bills, dinner, or a host of other mundane things. My mind would be wandering, and I couldn't focus it no matter how hard I tried. I would attempt to just silently chant the Reiki symbol names for the session, but still my mind would wander back to the mundane world. I grew angry at times because I had come to expect the visionary, but in the end, I was learning detachment. The sessions that were visionary for me were not necessarily the best sessions for my clients, and the sessions that were boring for me often led to some of the biggest breakthroughs for my clients. It wasn't about me, and it still isn't. I am not in charge, the universal life force is. I am the vessel for the energy, but it is not about my psychic gifts or lack thereof. If I need to see something or repeat it to a client, I trust that I will be told what I need to do. If I simply need to lay my hands on a person, then I focus on doing so, without any expectations. The ability to detach is the greatest gift I have received from Reiki. I have learned to have focus and intention, yet remain detached from the outcome. I have then been able to apply this powerful wisdom to my magickal practice.

Money and Reiki

Money is one of the most controversial issues in the Reiki world. Some practitioners charge for sessions and classes, while others give them for free. And there are a host of other arrangements in between that people have created for Reiki.

The problem arises when one person disagrees with another's method of exchange. Some practitioners in the most traditional schools of Reiki in the West charge vast sums of money, in the neighborhood of ten thousand dollars for Reiki Mastership. Many modern Western Reiki Masters felt that was too high a sum and went "independent," or rogue, from the Usui tradition, and set fees that they felt were more reasonable. Some teachers took it a step further and felt that everyone has a right to Reiki and should get it for free. Each perspective has its merits, and I can't judge if anyone is right or wrong completely.

When I started on a traditional Usui Reiki path, I was told that the high fees are a sign of respect and exchange. I was reminded of the story of Dr. Usui and how one must value these gifts. We must honor the teachers, and one of the ways we exchange energy in this society is through currency. Currency is simply a form of energy, like stored ki, and in the modern world, exchanging currency is more practical than becoming a house servant to a master. I agreed and had no problem with this. As for the Reiki Master fees, to become a teacher, I was told, requires a full-time commitment. The high fee is to show you are serious about dedicating your life to Reiki and not just doing it part-time. If you want to do Reiki part-time, then be a Reiki One or Two practitioner. If you want to dedicate yourself to it, and it becomes the most important thing to you, then you can acquire the class fee. The fee discourages those who are not serious. Not knowing any more, I had to agree.

Then I was introduced to a circle of independent Reiki Masters, those who have broken away from the Usui tradition, or those taught by other independents, mostly in a form of the Tibetan traditions of Reiki. They suggested that such fees were not reasonable, and that Reiki should be available to everyone. Fees should be set accordingly. Some set lower fees, while others barter or have a sliding scale. Such independents believed that Reiki was high priced due to either cultural misunderstanding or greed. One folk tale says that Takata claimed that Americans would not value Reiki if it was not expensive, so they must "pay through the nose." Although that story circulates, there is equally compelling anecdotal evidence that Takata didn't want to charge such high rates, but had similar experiences to Dr. Usui when she did not. I'm not sure how such high fees became the norm.

The last category is free Reiki for everyone. This is a marvelous sentiment, but I have to admit, like Usui and perhaps Takata, I too have had less than stellar experiences giving free sessions and healings. Since metaphysical healing and teaching has become my full-time profession, I've struggled with the issue of charging, but it has become a necessity with the demands placed on my time. I could not support myself otherwise.

If something is spiritual, should you charge for it? I think everyone has to answer this question personally. I paid to receive my Reiki training, and it was life-changing. I also paid for my college degree, music lessons, art lessons, and horseback riding lessons, which were also life-changing. They were also spiritual, yet not as mystical or quasi-religious as Reiki. You could argue that Reiki is not a religion, and therefore there is no ethical problem with charging for it. I've decided to follow the example of my teachers whom I respect and charge similar rates for similar services, but remain flexible as needs arise. For a while I had a sliding scale, suggesting a price range and letting people pay what they could afford. Although that worked well sometimes, many people complained about it. They felt uncomfortable choosing the price, and said that any other service has a set price, and suggested I do the same. Few massage therapists or massage therapy schools have a sliding scale.

I know the only reason I took Reiki Two from my teacher, Joanna, and was inspired by her to continue, was because she came highly recommended and the price was reasonable, since I was unemployed at the time. I met another highly regarded Reiki teacher who charged much more, but opted for Joanna. Now, some people think my prices are cheap, while others think they are expensive. It depends on what you are expecting, but very few have left my classes feeling that they did not get what they paid for in terms of a professional, well-taught, experiential class. They are not paying for the Reiki energy or even the attunement, but for my time, effort, writing, and guidance. They are paying for the structured experience of the class, rather than the energy of Reiki.

One technique that some independent Reiki Masters are using is charging the same amount, but in different currencies. One tradition charges three hundred for Reiki One, five hundred for Reiki Two, and ten thousand for Reiki Teacher level. They equate the numbers with a unit of energy, of ki. Any currency unit can be a value of ki. So instead of ten thousand dollars, it could be ten thousand quarters, dimes, or pennies. The value could even be ten thousand pesos! A few teachers exchange time, not money, with their students. Students agree to either work in the Reiki teacher's clinic or exchange their own professional services with the teacher. My friend Michelle asks recipients of treatments to "pay it forward" like the movie of the same name, having the person promise to help another as payment.

Those involved in the free Reiki movement often have practices that are not as structured. Most teach informally, one on one with friends and acquaintances. "Free" Reiki teachers feel the others are trying to control and profit from something that should be shared by all. They freely give attunements, but some do not give any real training or teach the history, so we have a lot of Reiki practitioners who cannot really even define what Reiki is or how it works, creating a lot of fallacies. Some teach online through distance attunements.

People will find the right teachers and students to match their own needs and learning. Teachers learn just as much from class experience as students do, if not more. If the situation is not right and it is not serving a purpose, then people will stop coming to the classes.

Money is a sensitive issue in most matters, and it can provoke some strong reactions in us. I know it did, and still does, for me. Seek to learn from your reactions and patterns around money, and do as your higher guidance directs.

Reiki and the Law

The future of Reiki and the law is murky for me. I have no idea in what direction it will head. I hope for a world with the freedom to do Reiki as needed, without hassles, but can also understand the importance of helping consumers know who is qualified and who is not. But who determines that? Right now, it's a local issue, though prior to this writing I became aware of various bills to put the Reiki Alliance or various massage associations in charge in certain locations. But to my knowledge, none have passed.

The first issue at hand is the legality of touch. Most people in our society who touch others for a living are often licensed to touch. Most Reiki practitioners have no state recognition, so they do not have a license to touch. But, unlike massage therapists and other body workers, there is no physical manipulation of tissue involved in Reiki. You simply rest your hands on the person. Still, that brings up issues of body privacy and gender for some.

The sensitivity of this issue can vary from location to location. I reside in New Hampshire, whose state motto is "Live free or die." The political scene in New Hampshire is usually pretty conservative, but for once that has worked in my favor, because no one seems to be that concerned about touching someone during Reiki as long as everyone is upfront and understands what is involved. Most are more worried that Reiki is a New Age sham or cult, but feel if people want to spend their money on it, it's a free country. But when attending a Reiki share clinic in Massachusetts, I had the organizer scream at me when I placed my hands on the recipient, "What are you doing?!? I don't know what you are doing, but we do REIKI here, nothing else!" Apparently she had only learned "no contact" Reiki, where you place your hands above a person, but never touch. I teach my students that method as an alternative for some sensitive people, but not as the preferred method. She found it hard to believe that Reiki was originally a hands-on healing form. I feel touch is an integral part of Reiki healing, since so many people in need of healing do not receive healthy touch regularly in their lives.

One legal option in this situation is a disclaimer or disclosure form. Although not necessarily a binding agreement, if you provide in writing what occurs in a session and have someone sign off on it, then you can theoretically prove that everything was explained if anyone has a complaint.

Besides the issue of inappropriate touch, either that which is sexual or injurious, most courts also want to ensure that Reiki practitioners are not practicing medicine without a license. With that in mind, I tell all my students to never diagnose an illness and never prescribe a medical course of action. I present Reiki as a complement to other forms of healthcare, whether allopathic or homeopathic. No matter how psychically sure you are of a diagnosis, always phrase it as a suggestion. Don't say, "You have liver cancer." Say, "Intuitively, I feel there is some malignancy in the liver. I highly suggest you have a medical professional assess it." Don't tell anyone to stop taking their medication, or change the dosage, no matter how psychically sure you are. Suggest that they consult with their healthcare practitioner. You may be surprised to know that some doctors are willing to consider this information. I have a client who takes heavy doses of psycho-pharmaceuticals, and after a session, I told her that my guidance said it was time to change the balance of medications. Her doctor actually agreed, and became interested in her "alternative" techniques of healing.

Another defense is to become ordained as a minister. I am ordained for other reasons, because it is helpful to have legal recognition since I am considered a High Priest in the pagan community. I can perform legal weddings, enter intensive-care units, and make prison visits under the auspices of clergy. But when someone comes to me for healing and Reiki, they know I am doing it under a spiritual, mystical umbrella, and there is no illusion about it being traditional medicine. Legally, ministers are allowed to touch clients as a part of spiritual counsel and healing, so I am protected. Though I am thankful for this protection, I don't anticipate needing to call on it anytime soon. If you are more strongly associated with the medical aspects of Reiki and practice it professionally, you might want to look into getting practitioner's insurance. Some Reiki organizations provide such services to members.

The next legal issue is the standards and ethics of a Reiki practitioner. There are no set standards in the Reiki world, though many guilds, associations, and traditions pass along their own personal ethics. None are necessarily legally enforceable, but are points of common courtesy and respect among clients and practitioners. Some key points include making the client feel comfortable, providing a description of what will occur during a session, keeping information confidential, and respecting boundary issues. You can share information with your teacher or another practitioner in a clinical way, if you are having difficulties, but do so without sharing names or personal information. Integrity is everything.

If you choose to open a professional Reiki practice, check with your state and local governments to see if there are any regulations or concerns you should be aware of before starting.

The last legal hurdle is by far the silliest. I call it the ™ Wars, or Trademark Wars. The Trademark Wars are the bids to trademark and control the various "new" traditions of Reiki, to regulate who can teach it, how you teach it, what manuals you use, and ultimately who is in charge of any changes. I can understand the desire to maintain standards and make sure a tradition doesn't veer too far from its origins, but some methods are just so contrary to what I learned Reiki to be about. But granted, I adopted the ethics of my independent Reiki Master and relish my independence.

If we are really using these ancient principles and tapping into a universal life force, can we trademark it? Yes, we can trademark the system, but we cannot trademark wisdom, and that is what will float to the top in any tradition, leaving the rest behind. The symbols can't really be trademarked. Notice how many show up in a variety of traditions.

No one can trademark the Bible or the Vedas. No one can trademark yoga or karate. Different movements and traditions can begin, but eventually they take on a life of their own, beyond the reach of their founder. The same is true with Reiki.

Again, the law, fallacies, and zealousness will hopefully fall away to the healing, love, and wisdom Reiki has to offer. If I have a vision for the future of Reiki, I see it becoming one of the rich magickal traditions of the next century, bridging the gap between East and West, surrender and true will. It has taught me so much as a magickal practitioner, and I hope I have brought something back to it, a new perspective. I hope to see Reiki grow and reach and transform, season to season, age to age, like the great tree of life itself.

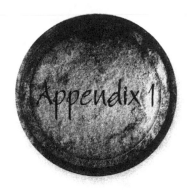

Appendix 1

Additional Reiki Symbols

At one time I was extremely preoccupied with learning all the symbols found in the various traditions of Reiki. Having found such a personal empowerment in other magickal symbols, the concept of Reiki symbols was a powerful step for me. I got caught up in the search for new symbols, rather than the healing and spiritual empowerment that comes with them. So instead of filling this entire book with all the symbols I have discovered and used, I opted to put them in an appendix. Many are symbols that I received from my guides during my initiations, while others are symbols that other Reiki practitioners have shared with me. When possible, I have listed the source of the symbol.

By no means is this a comprehensive list of the symbols used in the various Reiki traditions. I don't think anyone could compile a complete codex of symbols. Reiki is always evolving and transforming, like any spiritual tradition. If you want to work deeply with symbols, when you have a need, sit and meditate, and ask the energy of Reiki to give you a symbol to transform and heal your need. Some teachers claim that only special people—spiritual masters and gifted psychics—can bring through powerful symbols, and that's true. We are all special people. We are all masters, on all levels, waiting to remember our mastery. And we all have access to these healing gifts.

Al Luma

This symbol came to me to help clients hear messages and tune into guidance from spiritual beings during a healing session. It helps people who are too grounded in the body and fidgety to release and be in the moment, going with whatever experience occurs, without judgment. My guides called it a "cosmic ark," helping users travel. When I have used it, clients have reported that they were able to journey inward, visit spirit guides, and retrieve guidance when previously they were not able to do so.

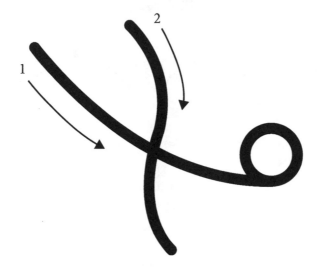

Figure 56: Al Luma

Anesthesia

This symbol was received by Shamballa Reiki Master-Teacher Susan Isabel of New Hampshire. Once drawn over the client, the symbol takes on a three-dimensional shape. Practitioners slowly push the symbol into the body to ease and numb pain. Note that the "petals" are drawn with an infinity-loop motion. The six petals are created by three infinity loops.

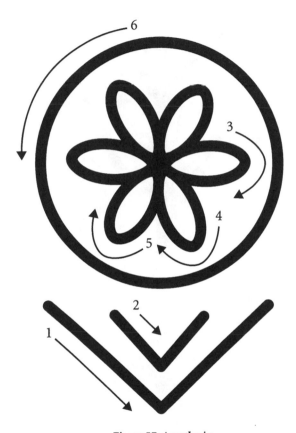

Figure 57: Anesthesia

Anti-Bacterial

Tired of relying on antibiotics prescribed by my doctor, yet having no luck with holistic medications, I asked the Reiki energy for aid in healing what I felt was a tonsil infection. I saw this symbol and used it repeatedly on my throat and chest and recovered much more quickly from my yearly throat infection.

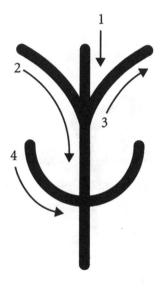

Figure 58: Anti-Bacterial

Anti-Burn

This symbol is used to reduce and heal damage caused by fire or chemical burns. It is put into the injured area, where it absorbs all heat to reduce the burning.

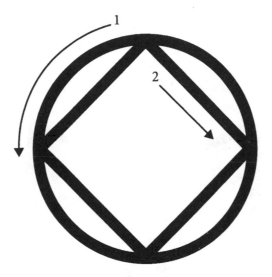

Figure 59: Anti-Burn

Anti-Poison

I received this symbol when I asked the Shamballa energy for a symbol to deal with poisons and toxins. I have an allergy to certain spider bites. Spider is one of my totems, and they show up in my life when I'm ignoring a message. When I've really been ignoring it, I've been bitten. When I was last bitten, I used this symbol repeatedly and the inflamed bump shrunk down to the size of a pimple, the itching went away, and there was no pain. For me, this symbol is incredibly healing, allowing me to get the message and not deal with the effects of the bite for weeks later.

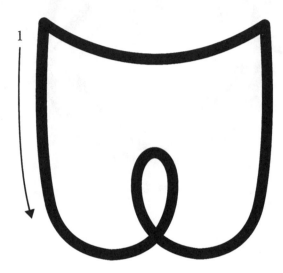

Figure 60: Anti-Poison

At Mata

At Mata is a symbol I received to help people cross over into a new threshold of healing. It is a gateway to open to a new, healthy, balanced you. At Mata helps remove emotional blocks that prevent you from seeing clearly.

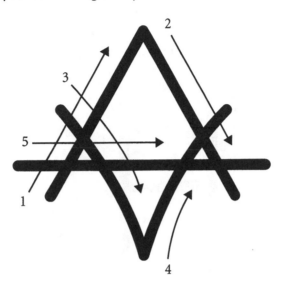

Figure 61: At Mata

Cellular Healing

The Cellular Healing symbol was received by my friend Kat Coree of Massachusetts when receiving a healing session with me. She saw it coming out of my hands, and every time she saw it, she got a message. She tells me that it allows the cells to "speak" directly to you, to understand and release cellular trauma. It also helps you understand and resolve previous actions—karma—that led you to an illness or injury. This symbol reminds me of the astrological symbol of Saturn (♄), the planet of karma.

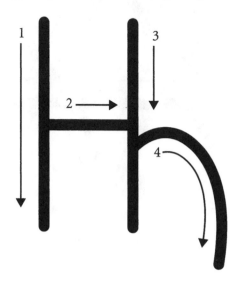

Figure 62: Cellular Healing

Dagu

Use this symbol to soften masculine energy when it is overabundant. It is for those who are overly aggressive, logical, or task/goal-oriented, while disregarding their feelings, emotions, intuition, and process. It heals male energy to honor all aspects of the self and balances warrior energy to be the spiritual warrior, the keeper of peace, rather than the aggressor. I received this symbol when personally working on the spiritual warrior path.

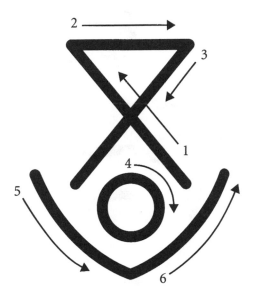

Figure 63: Dagu

Dai Koko Mi

I received this symbol and was told by my guides that it is a Master symbol to be used only in healing initiations. Dai Koko Mi cleanses the chakras and opens each center. The seven strokes are symbolic of the seven main chakras. I must admit that I don't use this symbol very often, and prefer the traditional Di Ko Mio.

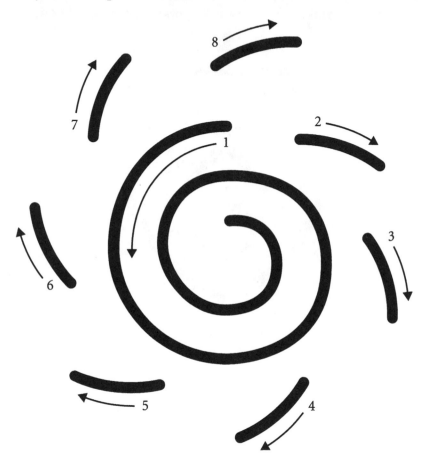

Figure 64: Dai Koko Mi

Dazu

While walking a dog in New Hampshire, I received this symbol for aligning with, and healing on, the devic (nature spirit) level. Use it anytime you are in nature. I draw it over plants after I harvest them for magickal and medicinal purposes. It is not a specific Earth healing symbol, but it helps provide individual healing and wholeness to nature spirits, devas, plants, and minerals. It eases any disturbances in the natural world created by humans. I even use it on my houseplants.

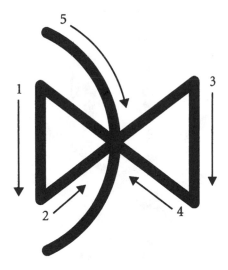

Figure 65: Dazu

Dragonfly

This symbol is used to break through the illusion of life and see clearly. It calls upon dragonfly animal medicine. When used on the throat, it helps you speak without illusions. It also helps you connect to your inner child. This symbol was received by Jessica Arsenault, United Kingdom.

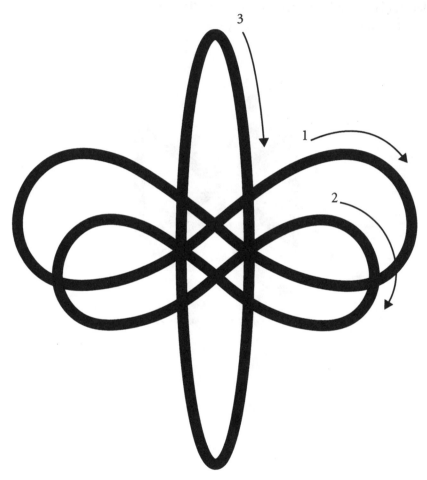

Figure 66: Dragonfly

Energy Gatherer

This symbol is used during planetary alignments. It creates compassion for the Earth. This symbol was channeled by Loril Moondream. She received this information to describe the symbol: "Envisioning the future of the Earth."

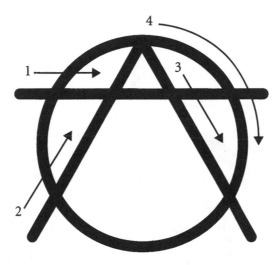

Figure 67: Energy Gatherer

Harmony

Harmony balances the power brought in by a healing session. It balances the flow and polarity of any energy inside the body and the aura. Harmony seals and protects, like Cho Ku Rei, and can be used at the end of a session to regulate the new energies within the body. It is the first symbol I received, at my Reiki Two initiation.

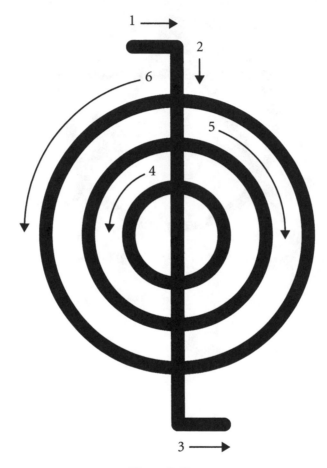

Figure 68: Harmony

Kir Mall

Use this "cure-all" symbol to relieve pain and discomfort when you cannot take the time to sit and meditate. The four loops balance the four elements within you. I received this symbol.

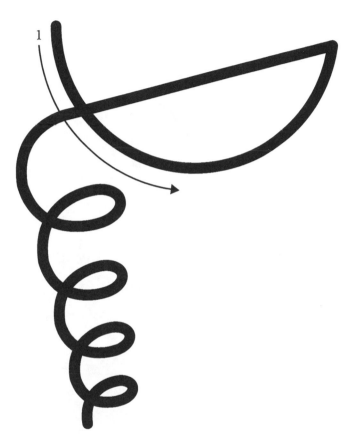

Figure 69: Kir Mall

Kundalini Balance

This symbol activates and balances kundalini force, the energy of awareness. It clears the kundalini channels between chakras to prepare for the smoother flow of energy during a session and as consciousness raises in everyday life. I received this symbol.

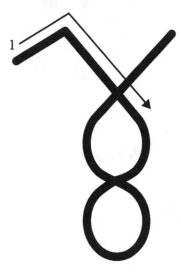

Figure 70: Kundalini Balance

Live Li

This is one of my favorite symbols that I have received. Live Li is similar to Motor Zanon, but it is used to remove all kinds of unwanted energy, not just virus particles. When drawn above the body and then "pushed in," it creates a three-dimensional tetrahedron with a mouth-like opening. This shape travels through the body, devouring any harmful, unbalanced energy and breaking up dense energies. Chant "Live Li" three times when putting it into the body. Chant "Li Live" three times when calling it out of the body.

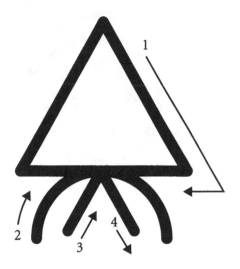

Figure 71: Live Li

Luma

This symbol is used to align feminine cycles and align with the cycles of the universe. It brings you back into balance with nature. The chaneller of this symbol is unknown, but it is shared by Shamballa Master-Teacher Phyllis Brooks, MA.

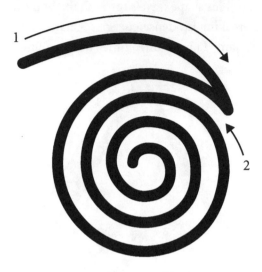

Figure 72: Luma

Perfect Love and Trust

Use this symbol to inspire love and trust. This symbol was received by Reiki Master and Shamballa Master-Teacher Jamie Gallant, NH.

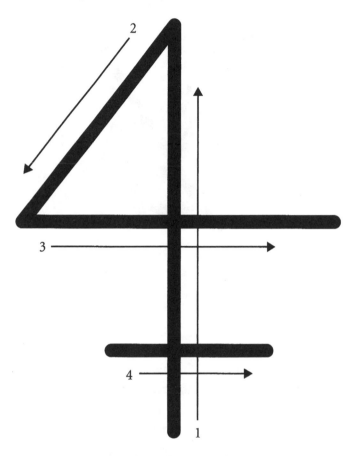

Figure 73: Perfect Love and Trust

Ra Ta Rio

This symbol integrates opposing identities and self-images, helping one make peace with the shadow self and face fear about death and mortality. I received this symbol.

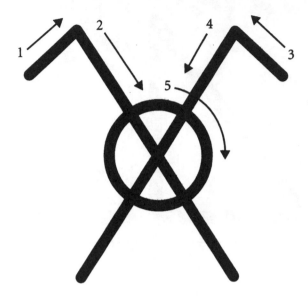

Figure 74: Ra Ta Rio

Third Eye Memory

Use this symbol before a meditation or journey to help you recall and understand any information you are given. This symbol was received by Derek O'Sullivan, MA.

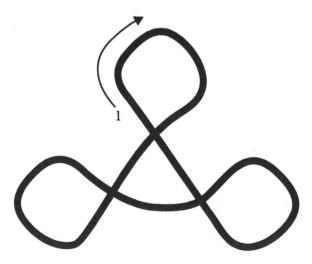

Figure 75: Third Eye Memory

Um Mal

Use this symbol to reconnect the physical aspects of the self with the spiritual aspects. It is for those who have a physical lifestyle that is in conflict with their spiritual beliefs. Um Mal allows one access to deep-seated emotions and fears to be brought up and healed. It helps one dive deep into repressed areas for conscious exploration. I received this symbol.

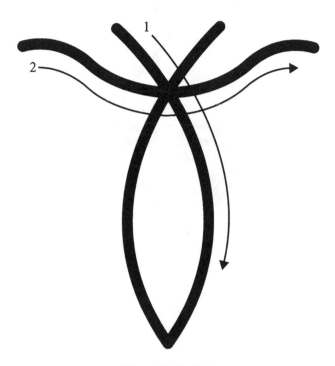

Figure 76: Um Mal

Walking on Air

This symbol is used to help you rise above and bring lightness to your walk, keeping you from feeling trapped by the problems of the world. This symbol was received by Susan Isabel, NH.

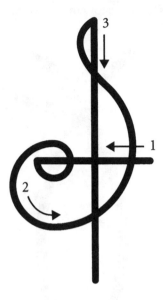

Figure 77: Walking on Air

Why Ti

This symbol integrates new energy and higher frequencies into the body. It helps balance the chakras when drawn from crown to root. It also helps one be more open and accepting of change. I received this symbol.

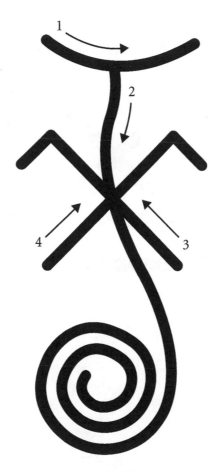

Figure 78: Why Ti

Zen Lu Ma

Use Zen Lu Ma to break apart tough mental or emotional blocks, or physical blocks and pains in the body. Once drawn, this symbol will take on a spinning action and enter the body to remove blocks. I received this symbol.

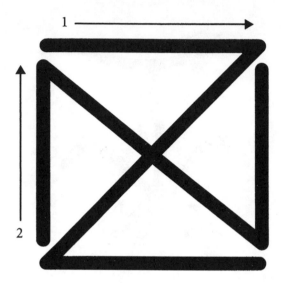

Figure 79: Zen Lu Ma

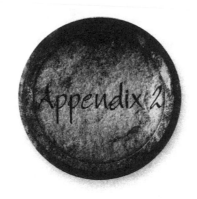

Reiki Herbal

Use this as an introduction to the magickal and spiritual properties of plants. In no way is this a complete magickal or medicinal herbal. Use it as a springboard, but always consult a reputable medicinal herbal or professional herbalist before consuming any herbs internally. Seek out a reputable aromatherapy resource before using aromatherapy for medicinal uses. Many magickal herbs are poisonous, and other usually benign plants can be toxic in certain forms, particularly essential oils.

Anise: The various forms of anise are used in love magick and to develop psychic ability. Star anise is my favorite. The star form, used whole, is quite magickal. It makes a wonderful charm.

Basil: Basil as a flower essence or plant spirit medicine is used for balancing sexuality, sexual energy, and identity. It can be used in love and lust magick, as well as for physical fertility. The essential oil's scent keeps one present in the moment.

Cinnamon: Cinnamon is a wonderful spice used for flavoring. Magickally, it is used for protection and prosperity. Burning cinnamon clears unwanted energy and creates a sacred space. In potions and charms, it is used for money magick, expanding your resources. Cinnamon plant spirit medicine helps warm the body and spirit.

Clover, Red: Red clover is another wonderful herb, used in magick and healing. A traditional love and prosperity herb, its spirit medicine helps balance feminine energies.

Cloves: Another spice, cloves can also be used for protection and prosperity. Whole clove spikes are used as a substitute for nails in protection and binding spells.

Comfrey: Comfrey's magick is in building. The herb builds connective tissues. Spiritually, it is used for grounding, building, and reconnecting. Comfrey flower essence can be used to reconnect to memories, particularly past-life memories. Ruled by the planet Saturn, comfrey can also be used for protection.

Dandelion: As an herb, dandelion root is used for the liver. Spiritually, the liver is where we store anger, so dandelion magick can be used to heal anger and find a healthy way to express it. Dandelion is also used for prosperity magick, grounding, and transformation, as the flower transforms into silky light seeds.

Frankincense: Frankincense is a golden resin that was highly valued in the ancient world. As an herb of the Sun, it is used for healing, inspiration, peace, and prosperity. When burned, the vibration of the incense creates sacred space, banishing all harm.

Garlic: Garlic is a very protective herb, as our legends tell us to use it to ward off ghouls and vampires. Garlic's spirit expels unwanted energies and prevents new unwanted energies from attaching, like a psychic repellant. Garlic as food, flower essence, infused oil, or spirit medicine confers this protection.

Hawthorn: Hawthorn is used herbally for the heart and circulatory system. Mystically, the hawthorn opens, heals, and protects the heart. The spikes on the tree represent the power of protection.

Lavender: Lavender is a wonderful, versatile herb. The essential oil can bring peace in small quantities, or stimulate in larger amounts. Magickally, the herb is used for peace and spirituality, meditation, psychic development, protection, and communication.

Lemon: The energy of lemon is cooling and watery, awakening psychic ability. It helps the user tune in to the emotional body and heal any repressed traumas.

Lemon Balm: Lemon balm is one of my favorite herbs. Medicinally, I use the tea and tincture to soothe the nerves, calm the stomach, and generally bring a clear head to any difficult situations. Magickally, it opens the gates to spiritual communication and psychic ability.

Motherwort: Motherwort is an herb of the Goddess. Medicinally and spiritually, it aids women in all times of life. Magickally, motherwort is for connecting to the Goddess, regardless of your gender, and is used in love and fertility magick.

Mugwort: Mugwort is a very potent magickal herb used for Moon magick. Named for the moon goddess Artemis, the entire artemesia family of herbs is very powerful. Mugwort can be used herbally for relaxation, but in magick it is used for dreams, prophecy, psychic ability, and astral travel. It makes a great incense.

Nettles: Nettles, or stinging nettle, is an herb of protection, fire, and the warrior. It has its own built-in mechanism—stingers. Medicinally, nettles are a great cure-all when you don't know what is wrong, particularly for the nervous system.

Myrrh: Myrrh is another of my favorite herbs. Myrrh is associated with the Moon and Saturn and used in protection magick and psychic work. I love to use it in conjunction with frankincense, since frankincense embodies the masculine and myrrh embodies the feminine. As an incense, it is a powerful cleanser and protector.

Oak: Oak is a powerful tree, associated with Celtic magick. The oak is associated with the Druids, as it is the tree of life and death. Oak bark, leaves, and, in particular, acorns are used in magick for protection, abundance, and fertility. A traditional protection spell calls for an acorn on every door frame and windowsill.

Oats: Oats and all grains are sacred to the Goddess of the Earth. They are nutritive, nourishing the body and the soul. Oats and oat straw soothe the nervous system. Magickally, they are used to soothe, nourish, connect to the goddess, and increase anything. They are a symbol of fertility and prosperity.

Patchouli: Patchouli is used for both protection and love magick. The strong earthy smell helps ground. The essential oil is a powerful way to evoke the power of patchouli.

Peppermint: Peppermint is an herb of the planet Mercury, and is used for clearing the mind and for communication. Medicinally, it soothes stomachaches.

Raspberry: Raspberry naturally resonates with the power of the Goddess, and can be used in healing all feminine issues. Medicinally, it is used for feminine reproductive healing. Magickally, it is used in love and fertility magick.

Rose: Rose is by far one of my favorite plants. Rose magick is for love, but all types of love, from romantic to spiritual love. The scent of rose uplifts the spirits. Rose spirit opens and heals the heart chakra.

Rowan: Rowan is a tree of protection. Its twigs and berries are used to protect one from harm, particularly from harmful magick. Rowan is a tree of witches, but ironically, according to traditional lore, rowan protects you from witchcraft.

Sage: The many plants that carry the name sage have protective properties. Garden sage, brush sage, and white sage are all burned and smudged to cleanse and purify a space. Sage is used in many Native American traditions.

Vervain: Vervain is a magickal all-purpose herb used for protection, purification, love, psychic ability, and power. Traditional lore usually refers to European or white vervain, though my magickal experiences with vervain have been with blue vervain, which is also used for communication and clarity.

Watermelon: The spirit of watermelon is used for conception and pregnancy. I've used the flower essence quite successfully for women seeking conception. Watermelon is also used in the magick of the Goddess and for symbolic fertility, for those seeking artistic or financial fertility.

Yarrow: Medicinally, yarrow can be used to stop bleeding. Spiritually, it heals rips and tears in the aura and energy body. It is an herb of protection, but is also aligned with the energy of movement and flow, like blood, and can be used in love magick.

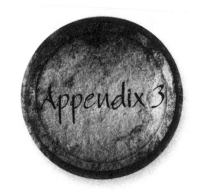

Color Magick

The following are some traditional magickal associations of colors. Use them for candle magick, charms, visualization, and symbols. Use them to determine the properties of plants and stones, but also follow your own intuition. Your personal connection to color can be different from tradition. You can also use your knowledge of the chakras to guide you in color magick.

Red	Energy, passion, stimulation, lust, protection, aggression, warrior
Red-orange	Critical intense healing, energy
Orange	Strong healing, energy, strength, willpower, mental clarity, memory, logic, knowledge
Gold	God energy, unconditional love, divine will, power, wealth, health
Yellow	Spirituality, communication, thoughts, logic, health, clarity
Green	Healing, love, growth, life, Mother Earth, prosperity, money, fertility
Turquoise	Higher love, higher heart, unconditional acceptance, divinity, balance
Blue	Peace, prosperity, spirituality, dreams, spirit healing

Pink   Love, happiness, self-esteem, romance

Indigo   Psychic energy, visualization, opening the senses

Purple   Spirituality, tranquility, balance

Violet   Cleansing, neutralization, balance, divinity, psychic powers

White   Healing, love, connection to all, healing, all-purpose, banishing, protection

Black   Grounding, magick, meditation, mystery, crossroads, crone goddesses

Brown   Healing, grounding, healing animals, stability

Rust   Removing unwanted energies, release, cleansing

Silver   Goddess energy, moon, maiden, emotional healing, psychic powers, cycles, fertility

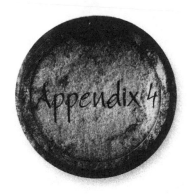

Quick Reference for Healing Symbols

Below is a list of potential issues and situations, along with potentially corresponding healing symbols. By no means is this list complete, as each symbol has a variety of uses and our knowledge of them grows as we use them. Each situation is different, so you will have to follow your own divine guidance to see if a particular symbol is relevant to the situation at hand.

Abuse

Addictions

Trauma

Unconscious Mind

Viral Infections

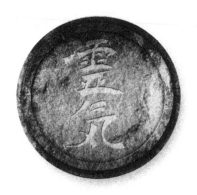

Bibliography

Amador, Vincent. *Karuna Ki: A Comprehensive Manual of the History, Practices, Symbols and Attunements of the Art of Karuna Ki.* An e-book. http://angelreiki.nu/karunaki. 1999–2001.

———. *Reiki Plain and Simple: A Comprehensive Guide to Usui Shiki Ryoho.* An e-book and comprehensive manual and articles on Reiki and Usui/Tibetan Reiki. http://angelreiki.nu. 1998–2001.

———. *Reiki Xtras: Additional Practices in Using Reiki or "Using Reiki That Is Not Usui Reiki."* An e-book. http://angelreiki.nu/xtras/ReikiXtras.htm. 1999–2001.

Anderson, Kathryn, and Gisele King. *Magnified Healing Celebration Manual.* Miami, FL: Magnified Healing, 1994.

———. *Magnified Healing Teaching Manual.* Miami, FL: Magnified Healing, 1992.

Barnett, Libby, and Maggie Chambers, with Susan Davidson. *Reiki Energy Medicine: Bringing Healing Touch into Home, Hospital, and Hospice.* Rochester, VT: Healing Arts Press, 1996.

Hensel, Thomas A., and Dr. Kevin Ross Emery. *The Lost Steps of Reiki: The Channeled Teachings of Wei Chi.* Portsmouth, NH: Lightlines Publishing.

Milner, Kathleen. *Reiki & Other Rays of Touch Healing*. Mesa, AZ: K. A. Milner, 1995.

―――. *Tera, My Journey Home: Seichem, Shamanism, Symbology, Herbs & Reincarnation*. Mesa, AZ: K. A. Milner, 1997.

Petter, Frank Arjava. *Reiki Fire: New Information about the Origins of the Reiki Power*. Twin Lakes, WI: Lotus Light Publications, 1997.

Pinney, Joanna. *Heart Light Reiki Master Teacher Guide to Usui-Tibetan Enhanced Reiki III Manual*. 1998.

Rand, William L. *Advanced Reiki Training Manual*. Southfield, MI: The Center for Reiki Training, 1996.

―――. *Reiki Three Manual*. Southfield, MI: The Center for Reiki Training, 1996.

Shewmaker, Diane Ruth. *All Love: A Guidebook for Healing with Sekhem-Seichim-Reiki and SKHM*. Beaverton, OR: Celestial Wellspring, 2000.

Stein, Diane. *Essential Reiki: A Complete Guide to an Ancient Healing Art*. Freedom, CA: Crossing Press, 1995.

Additional Online Resources

www.angelreiki.nu, *Reiki Plain and Simple*.

www.angelfire.com/mb/manifestnow/bluestar.html, *Higher Energy Systems and Metaphysical Healing*.

www.geocities.com/HotSprings/9434/branches1.html#RP, *Branches or Schools of Reiki*.

www.mahatma.co.uk, *Shamballa Multidimensional Healing*.

www.celestialwellspring.com, *Diane Ruth Shewmaker and Sekhem-Seichim-Reiki*.

www.skhm.org, *SKHM/Seichim*.

www.trtai.org, *Radiance Technique®*.

www.magnifiedhealing.com, *Magnified Healing*.

www.kathleenmilner.com/, *Kathleen Ann Milner and Tera Mai™*.

www.reiki.org, *William Lee Rand and The International Center for Reiki Training*.